Winning
with
Diabetes

Winning
with
Diabetes

Inspiring Stories from Athletes
to Help You Thrive

Mark D. Corriere, MD
Rita R. Kalyani, MD, MHS
Patrick J. Smith

Illustrated by Jennifer E. Fairman, CMI, FAMI

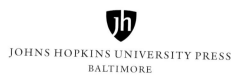

JOHNS HOPKINS UNIVERSITY PRESS
BALTIMORE

Note to the reader: This book is not meant to substitute for medical care of people with diabetes, and treatment should not be based solely on its contents. Instead, treatment must be developed in a dialogue between the individual—or the individual's parent—and their physician. Our book has been written to help with that dialogue.

Johns Hopkins University Press
2715 North Charles Street
Baltimore, Maryland 21218
www.press.jhu.edu

Library of Congress Cataloging-in-Publication Data

Names: Corriere, Mark D. (Mark Dominic), author. | Kalyani, Rita Rastogi, author. | Smith, Patrick J. (Patrick Joseph), 1966–, author. | Fairman, Jennifer E., illustrator.
Title: Winning with diabetes : inspiring stories from athletes to help you thrive / Mark D. Corriere, MD, Rita R. Kalyani, MD, MHS, and Patrick J. Smith.
Description: Baltimore : Johns Hopkins University Press, [2023] | Series: A Johns Hopkins Press health book | Includes index. | Summary: "This unique book shares some of the common challenges and successes athletes have encountered while living with diabetes, inspiring readers to take control of their diabetes and thrive"— Provided by publisher.
Identifiers: LCCN 2022021483 | ISBN 9781421445571 (hardcover) | ISBN 9781421445588 (paperback) | ISBN 9781421445595 (ebook)
Subjects: LCSH: Diabetes—Popular works.
Classification: LCC RC660.4 .C67 2023 | DDC 616.4/62--dc23/eng/20220615
LC record available at https://lccn.loc.gov/2022021483

A catalog record for this book is available from the British Library.

Special discounts are available for bulk purchases of this book. For more information, please contact Special Sales at specialsales@jh.edu.

To my wife, Suzy,
and children—Dominic, Molly, Sam, and Tommy
—for their unwavering support and love
—*Mark D. Corriere*

To my husband, Sachin, and children, Shaan and Sonia,
who are my greatest joy and
whose unending resilience and determination
continue to inspire me each day
—*Rita R. Kalyani*

To my wife, Deborah Shaller,
whose patience, love, and wisdom
have brightened my world for a whole lot of years.
And to Philip Quarry, whose memory was never far away
throughout the writing of this book.
—*Patrick J. Smith*

Contents

Preface

The world population doubled between the years 1980 and 2020. But during those same years, the number of people around the globe living with diabetes quadrupled.

The World Health Organization estimates that more than 500 million people have diabetes. The epidemic isn't confined to one country or continent. Developing and wealthy nations alike have seen sharp increases in the incidence of type 2 diabetes among their citizens.

In the United States, the Centers for Disease Control and Prevention estimates that 37.3 million Americans—more than 1 in 10—have diabetes. More than 7 million people in the country have the disease and don't know it.

While ethnic and racial minorities in the United States are slightly more likely than whites to have diabetes, the disease cuts across socio-economic, sex, and age demographics: diabetes does not discriminate.

But the news isn't all bad.

In our medical practices, we see patients day in and day out who are not just managing their diabetes but are thriving with it. They're determined to live active, healthy, and long lives—something that, as recently as the 1980s, was much more difficult to do than it is today. Scientific, medical, and technological advances have made managing diabetes simpler than it used to be.

We wrote this book to learn more about how athletes manage diabetes. In our research, we spoke with 16 different athletes about their experiences with the disease. How does diabetes affect their training? Is it different on game days? The excitement of a game or a match or a meet can release a flood of adrenaline, which has a profound effect on blood sugar. How do they keep their blood sugar from skyrocketing in the heat of competition? How did they learn to manage the disease? These are only a few of the questions we asked. And each of the athletes in this book had answers that were unique to them.

When we talk about the growing epidemic of diabetes in the United States and around the world, approximately 90%–95% of cases are type 2 and up to 5% are type 1. Type 2 diabetes is most commonly diagnosed in adults who are obese and have other risk factors, such as a strong family history. We encountered few athletes with type 2 diabetes, given the intense exercise and training regimens that athletes often follow. In fact, every athlete in this book lives with type 1 diabetes, except for one who was diagnosed with type 2 diabetes soon after his professional career ended. Some were diagnosed when they were young children; others, like Olympic gold-medal swimmer Gary Hall Jr., were diagnosed as their athletic careers were just taking flight.

Our purpose in this book is to relate some of the common challenges and successes that these athletes have encountered while living with diabetes and to let people with diabetes know that you don't have to be a superstar elite athlete to thrive.

You'll read the stories they shared with us: stories of ups and downs, good days and bad days, elation and frustration. These athletes' stories dispute the idea that diabetes will beat you once you're diagnosed.

You'll read that it's not always easy. But one of the most important lessons sports teaches us is about bouncing back from a tough day. Even the greatest, winningest teams in history lost games once in a while. The legendary 1927 New York Yankees, with Babe Ruth and Lou Gehrig, lost 44 games on their way to winning the World Series. When Michael Jordan's Chicago Bulls beat the Seattle SuperSonics for the 1995–1996 NBA title, they had lost 10 regular-season games and two in the Finals.

There's no shame in losing. When our best effort isn't quite enough to push us across the finish line first, we congratulate the winner and start preparing for the next race or game or match. Part of that preparation is learning from our losses. What worked? What didn't? Do we need to make major adjustments? Or just a few tweaks?

When a basketball team's sharpshooter knocks down several three-point shots in a row, the opposing coach calls a time-out and the team regroups. How can they stop the shooter? Who can guard that shooter on defense? Do our opponents have any tendencies that we can exploit?

Consider this book a time-out.

Even if your diabetes is well-managed and under control, we hope our book helps you regroup and take inspiration, and maybe even a few pointers, from athletes who have the disease and who have spent lifetimes fine-tuning and incorporating their diabetes management into their athletic pursuits.

It's our hope that readers will gain a better understanding of diabetes, whether type 1 or 2, and, ultimately, will draw inspiration from at least one of the athletes in this book. The athletes with whom we spoke for this book were unfailingly generous with their time and were candid about their experiences with diabetes. Like everyone, they get discouraged or frustrated on days when, for whatever reason, blood sugar is just hard to control. But the determination and the drive that compels them to compete is exactly what they need to manage diabetes.

Some of the athletes in this book are professionals, some are amateurs. Some are retired, some are still actively competing. Some are pioneers in their sports. But each of them has had to make their diabetes care a top priority, not just to compete at elite levels but to stay healthy.

Despite our years in the field of endocrinology and diabetes, we were surprised by a theme that emerged during our interviews: more than a few of the athletes say they're successful not in spite of their diabetes but because of it.

Think of that for a moment.

They attribute their success to a chronic disease that needs attention multiple times a day, every day of their lives.

This book presents the stories the athletes told us, most of which are followed by our brief author commentary. Each chapter introduces a new topic or challenge that people with diabetes commonly face during their journey while living with the disease.

We sought a diverse group of athletes, including both men and women, to interview for this book. In addition to athletes of diverse racial and ethnic backgrounds, we included athletes varying in age from teenagers to older adults. They compete in many different sports and live in many different parts of the United States and the world. The athletes we interviewed and who are featured in this book are:

- *Mark Andrews*, professional American football player; tight end with the National Football League's Baltimore Ravens
- *Doug Burns*, American strength athlete, bodybuilder, and former Natural Mr. Universe
- *Lauren Cox*, American professional basketball player for the Women's Basketball League in Spain
- *Will Cross*, American mountain climber who summited Mount Everest, as well as the highest peaks on all seven continents and walked to both the North and South Poles
- *Adam Driscoll*, American cyclist and former member of a four-man relay team that rode in Race Across America, the world's longest bicycle race
- *Missy Foy*, American distance runner who twice qualified for the Olympic marathon trials
- *Gary Hall Jr.*, American swimmer and winner of five gold, three silver, and two bronze medals at the 1996, 2000, and 2004 Olympic Games
- *Kate Hall-Harnden*, American track and field athlete and national high school–record holder in the long jump and NCAA champion who previously qualified for the final at the United States Olympic Trials
- *Monique Hanley*, Australian cyclist who raced in Race Across America and previously cycled solo across Canada

- *Jason Johnson*, American former Major League Baseball pitcher
- *Charlie Kimball*, American race car driver competing in the IndyCar Series
- *Kylee Perez*, American softball player who played for the University of California, Los Angeles, and four-time All-Pac 12 player
- *Cathy and Riley Reese*, head coach and five-time national champion with the University of Maryland women's lacrosse team, and her son who now plays on the men's lacrosse team at the same college
- *Sébastien Sasseville*, Canadian mountain climber and distance runner who summited Mount Everest and ran across Canada
- *Scott Verplank*, American professional golfer who has played on the Professional Golfers Association (PGA) and PGA Champions tours
- *Dominique Wilkins*, American basketball Hall of Famer and vice president of basketball for the National Basketball Association's Atlanta Hawks

A few of the athletes we interviewed describe experimenting with their diabetes management in ways we do not necessarily recommend. It's important to follow your physician's advice when it comes to exercise and trying new things related to managing your diabetes. In other words, some of the content in this book falls into the "don't try this at home" category but nonetheless demonstrates the perseverance and determination of these athletes.

Thank you for reading. We hope you enjoy this book as much as we've enjoyed writing it.

Acknowledgments

This book would not have been possible without the generosity and time of the athletes that we interviewed and who shared their candid stories of living with diabetes: Mark Andrews, Doug Burns, Lauren Cox, Will Cross, Adam Driscoll, Missy Foy, Gary Hall Jr., Kate Hall-Harnden, Monique Hanley, Jason Johnson, Charlie Kimball, Kylee Perez, Cathy and Riley Reese, Sébastien Sasseville, Scott Verplank, and Dominique Wilkins. Thank you for your inspirational stories and commitment to the diabetes community.

Thanks are also due to Karen and David Nitkin, Jeff and Sonja Perez, Jelani Downing, Nicholas Argento, and Linell Smith.

We appreciate the contributions of the exceptionally talented Jennifer E. Fairman, CMI, FAMI, and her illustrations throughout this book.

We are particularly grateful for the guidance of our editor at Johns Hopkins University Press, Joe Rusko, whose input was critical at all stages.

We especially acknowledge our families for their patience and support as we worked on this book.

Finally, we are indebted to the many patients that we have had the privilege to care for and whose personal journeys of living with diabetes have shown us what it means to thrive with this disease.

Winning
with
Diabetes

Chapter 1

The Diagnosis of Diabetes

Why me?

GARY HALL JR. won two silver and two gold medals at the 1996 Summer Olympic Games in Atlanta. The 22-year-old swimmer was a favorite to bring home more gold from Sydney in 2000. But during his grueling training sessions, Hall began to notice his hands trembling at swim practice. He found that a few slugs of Gatorade would make the shakes go away.

"I wrote it off to fatigue," says Hall. "Training for the Olympics is intense. You expend an incredible amount of energy in a practice swim."

Hall also noticed that, lately, he felt thirsty all the time. "But I was training in Arizona," he says. "Everybody tells you, 'it's a dry heat.'" Everyone gets thirsty in the desert, right? More than once, Hall found himself in the grocery checkout line buying 6 gallons of various beverages and nothing else. "I'd go to the parking lot and chug half a gallon of whatever I bought."

But when he couldn't read traffic signs until his car was right in front of them, Hall wondered if something might be wrong. Though the Sydney games were only 18 months away, he took a break from training.

"I was in and out of bed for a couple of weeks," he says. "I thought it was some kind of flu or something. Or that I was just run-down from training so hard."

Despite weeks of near-constant rest, Hall's condition worsened. Eventually, even the simplest of tasks required two days in bed to recover.

"I'd eat something and feel so terrible I'd have to go back to bed."

Meanwhile, he'd also spent weeks dreading a party his then-girl-friend committed him to attending. A friend had gotten engaged, and Hall's girlfriend insisted he accompany her to the celebration. When the party date rolled around, Hall told her he didn't feel well.

"I remember telling her, 'I feel sick. Please, just go without me.'"

Not an option, she said.

Exhausted by this mystery condition, the Olympian struggled out of bed and expended nearly all his strength just to pull some clothes onto his body, which was suddenly 20 pounds lighter than only a few months before. Hall drove them to the party, protesting all the way that he felt lousy and wouldn't make for good company. His girlfriend still wasn't buying it.

When they arrived, Hall managed to drag himself out of the car, took a few steps, and collapsed in a heap on the ground.

"My vision went red, and I blacked out. I couldn't stand up." The girlfriend, still unconvinced, was furious that he'd go to such lengths to avoid this party. As she railed at him from the sidewalk, Hall crawled back to the car and climbed into the driver's seat.

Unwisely, he drove himself home and staggered back to bed. Confused and afraid, he called his father.

Gary Hall Sr. is himself a three-time Olympic medalist, compet-ing in the Mexico City, Munich, and Montreal Games. And, for 25 years, he practiced ophthalmology in Phoenix.

"In his practice, my dad saw a lot of people with diabetic retinop-athy," Hall says. "He was beginning to suspect I might have diabetes."

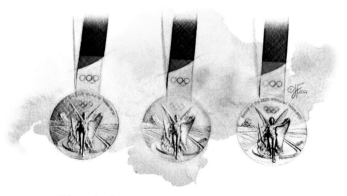

Olympic silver, gold, and bronze medals

Gary Senior accompanied his son to the family's general practitioner, who, after a brief exam, shared the father's suspicion of diabetes. When a finger-stick test came back with glucose levels of 300 mg/dl—much higher than normal—the doctor gave Gary Junior his first-ever injection of insulin. He also gave him the name and address of an endocrinologist, ordering him to get there immediately.

"We got over there, and the waiting room was packed," says Hall. "When it was finally my turn, the guy came in and told me, 'oh yeah, you have type 1 diabetes.' That was it. That was the whole diagnosis. He had one foot out the door and told me to see the nurse at the end of the hall."

That nurse, surrounded by mountains of brochures and leaflets explaining the basics of diabetes, talked to Hall about his diagnosis and what it meant.

But a scant 18 months before the Sydney Olympics, Hall had only one question: can I still compete?

The nurse's answer: no.

"She said I could swim for, like, recreation or for health," Hall recalls. "But nobody'd ever competed in anything like Olympic swimming with diabetes, she told me. That just wasn't going to be possible anymore."

A despondent Hall decided that a life without Olympic swimming wasn't worth living. He packed a bag for one last journey, this time to Costa Rica, where he planned to disappear forever.

Maybe it was the beauty of the Pacific Ocean. Maybe it was the seclusion of the Costa Rican beaches. But Hall, armed only with a few books about how to manage diabetes, decided to give life another go.

"Somehow, I found some solace down there and came to terms with diabetes," he says. "I thought maybe I could find a way to swim again."

— Expert Commentary —

When Gary Hall Jr. was told he had diabetes, unfortunately, the endocrinologist gave him the news without too much compassion. The nurse told him that he could never participate in the Olympics. This lack of empathy from his care team undoubtedly influenced his decision to seclude himself from the outside world while he learned to accept the diagnosis. If only he had known at that time that he wasn't alone.

According to the US Centers for Disease Control and Prevention (CDC), in 1958, fewer than 1% of Americans had diabetes. The nation has seen an increase in the incidence of the disease almost every year since, with an especially sharp rise beginning in the late 1990s. Today, one in 10 Americans lives with any type of diabetes. Though type 2 diabetes represents the majority of cases (around 90%–95%), rates of type 1 diabetes represent up to 5% of cases and are also increasing around the world.

Even more staggering, the CDC estimates that almost three times that many Americans have prediabetes. Prediabetes means that a person's blood glucose levels are elevated but not yet in the diabetes range. This condition puts individuals at risk of developing type 2 diabetes in the future if they don't dramatically change their lifestyle. This starts as the body becomes resistant to the insulin they produce. If left untreated, their pancreas may slowly make less insulin over time. People who are overweight, physically inactive, or who have family members with the disease are most likely to develop type 2 diabetes. With the right approach, however, type 2 diabetes can be prevented—and sometimes even reversed.

At present, type 1 diabetes cannot be reversed since it results from auto-immune destruction of the insulin-producing cells in the pancreas. Those who are diagnosed with it will need to manage the disease, usually with insulin, for the rest of their lives.

———————

LIKE HALL, SÉBASTIEN SASSEVILLE was diagnosed with type 1 diabetes at age 22. But unlike Hall, Sasseville's athletic career was a long way off. He minces no words about his abilities.

"I suck at sports," the Quebec native laughs. "I didn't play hockey, unlike almost everyone else in our town."

Sasseville's assessment of his athletic ability is understated. Among his accomplishments are summiting Mount Everest, completion of numerous Ironman Triathlons, and a seven-day foot race across the Sahara Desert.

He's best known for a 2014 run that aimed to bring attention to type 1 diabetes in his native Canada. In February of that year, Sasseville laced up his running shoes and took off west from the craggy North Atlantic shores of St. John's, Newfoundland, the easternmost point in North America. In November, he ran out of room at the Pacific Ocean, having completed a trans-Canadian route—the equivalent of 170 marathons.

Also, unlike Hall, when it comes to diabetes, Sasseville saw the writing on the wall for months before seeing a doctor.

"My younger brother has type 1," says Sasseville, who started showing symptoms as a student at Quebec's Collège Laval a few years after he'd left his tiny hometown of Saint-Patrice-de-Beaurivage. "He was diagnosed at about 14, around six years before my diagnosis."

Sasseville remembered his brother's symptoms and, after he'd had them himself for a while, he had an inkling he knew what would come next.

"I was eating a lot but losing weight," he says. "I thought, 'aw shoot.' I kind of knew what was going on."

He drove himself to the hospital and learned that, sure enough, like his brother, he would live the rest of his life with type 1 diabetes.

"Unless there's a cure," he adds, hopefully.

For his family's sake, Sasseville is glad his diagnosis came after he'd left home for college.

"I was living in an apartment. I had a job. I was putting myself through school," he says. His independence meant he'd have to manage diabetes by himself. But it also spared his parents the difficulty of helping another child through the early days of the disease. "I saw how tough my brother's diabetes was on my parents."

"When I found out I had it too, my reaction was, 'Oh God, I don't want to put my parents through that again.'"

The Sasseville family had a difficult time in the early days of Sébastien's brother's diagnosis, learning to cook new foods and waking up in the middle of the night to administer injections. So Sasseville learned to manage the condition largely on his own.

"Like a lot of 22-year-olds, I was at the pub a lot," he says. "But I stopped drinking and thought maybe I could, like, exercise instead and maybe eat healthier. I have a disease that's forcing me to be healthy. It could be a lot worse."

— Expert Commentary —

Type 1 diabetes carries a genetic risk. If your sibling has type 1 diabetes, like Sasseville, your lifetime risk of also developing type 1 diabetes is about 5%. If your mother has type 1 diabetes, your chance of developing the disease before age 25 is between 2% and 4%. The child of a father with type 1 diabetes has a 6% lifetime risk.

Other risk factors for type 1 diabetes include environment, such as where you live (the disease is more common in the Northern Hemisphere) and ethnicity (non-Hispanic whites have the highest risk). Type 1 diabetes is most commonly diagnosed during the elementary or middle school years, but it is also increasingly being diagnosed in adulthood.

Similar to type 1 diabetes, type 2 diabetes also carries a substantial genetic risk. If a parent, sibling, or child (any first-degree relative) has type 2 diabetes, you have a higher-than-average risk (40%–50%) of getting it too. In addition to genetics, risk factors for type 2 diabetes include age older than 45 years, being overweight or obese, not exercising regularly, and for women, a history of gestational diabetes (diabetes during pregnancy) or polycystic ovarian syndrome.

CHARLIE KIMBALL was well into his race-driving career at 22 years of age.

At 18, a year after his career began, he finished third overall in the Formula Ford US Series, winning twice and earning seven podium appearances. Before he turned 21, Kimball had raced open-wheel cars on many of the world's most storied tracks, including Donington Park, Zandvoort, the Silverstone Circuit, and Nürburgring.

"I fell in love with racing early in life," he says. He'd been around the sport long enough to know that there were lots of job opportunities in the sport besides just driving. One way or another, Kimball knew he'd be in the racing business. But his dream was to advance his fledgling driver career.

Kimball recalls sitting in the endocrinologist's office, learning

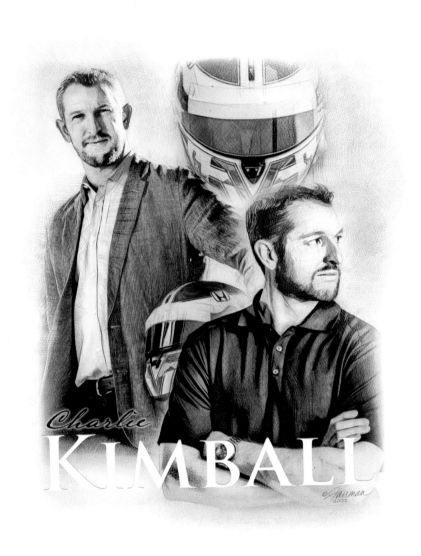

Charlie Kimball, American race car driver, competing in the IndyCar Series:
"Whether it was right after being diagnosed or the race just last weekend, I've learned something [about diabetes]."

his diagnosis of type 1 diabetes. A Southern California native and a Los Angeles Dodgers fan, he compares it to a big moment in a baseball game.

When he asked the doctor if he'd ever race again, Kimball recalls an interminable silence.

"It was a little like time slowed down. It felt like the defining play, the diving catch in the outfield in the World Series, when the whole stadium holds its breath."

While Kimball waited, the endocrinologist finished writing his notes, leaving a torturous pause.

"It seemed like forever, but it was probably three or four seconds."

At last, says Kimball, the doctor looked up from his notes and told him, "I don't see any reason why you can't. There are incredible people doing amazing things with diabetes all over the world. You may have to change how you go about it, but it shouldn't get in the way of you living your dreams."

At that moment, says Kimball, he decided to learn as much as he could about diabetes management.

"The motivator for me was to get back in the race car as soon as possible. I had a thirst and a curiosity to understand my diabetes. Since then, my life has been built around doing everything I possibly can to be successful on the racetrack."

— *Expert Commentary* —

Charlie Kimball was fortunate to have an endocrinologist who encouraged him to pursue his athletic aspirations and not let diabetes hold him back, demonstrating compassion in a manner that unfortunately Hall didn't benefit from in the early days of his diagnosis. Understanding the basics of glucose metabolism and insulin physiology was critical to Kimball's future success.

In many ways, sugar holds the keys to survival. A simple sugar called glucose supplies energy to living organisms' cells. Insulin is a hormone that acts as a fuel injector, permitting just as much glucose as our cells need to function.

Too much glucose and complications develop in the body. Too little glucose and the body, especially the brain, can't function. Kimball's type 1 diabetes means his body cannot produce insulin, leaving him without a way to regulate the glucose levels in his blood. When we eat, our bodies break the nutrients from food into various components that supply the nutrition we need to stay alive. After they're digested, carbohydrates and starches convert to monosaccharides, or single sugars, known as glucose. That glucose gets absorbed into our blood and is delivered to our cells.

Meanwhile, the pancreas—a roughly 6-inch organ that sits behind the stomach and beneath the right lobe of the liver—produces insulin. Because Kimball has type 1 diabetes, his pancreas does not produce insulin, and he relies on a synthetic version of the hormone that he must inject with a needle. Whether through a pen, a syringe, or attached to a small mechanical pump, the needle ideally delivers the exact dose of insulin that will regulate his blood glucose levels, properly fueling the billions of individual cells that make up his body.

The body can survive without any insulin for only a short time. Kimball's body would burn other fuels, such as protein and fat, until they were depleted. If this occurs for too long, acid can develop in the body, changing the pH and resulting in a life-threatening condition known as diabetic ketoacidosis. This causes serious illness or even death. In short, without insulin, Kimball's cells would go without nourishment, leading to the collapse of nearly every system in his body. His brain, muscles, nerves, cardiovascular system, and every other system that works in tandem to keep him healthy would eventually starve.

People with type 2 diabetes do produce insulin early in the course with the disease. However, their body is "resistant" to the insulin they are making and does not properly respond to it. This insulin resistance is the hallmark of type 2 diabetes and can be improved with exercise, weight loss, and medications. In patients with long-standing type 2 diabetes, their pancreas may reach a point where the insulin-producing cells (the beta cells of the pancreas) are no longer capable of making insulin. This leads to a combination of insu-

lin resistance and insulin deficiency. These patients require insulin therapy multiple times a day, similar to type 1 diabetes patients.

When glucose isn't properly regulated, it can lead to excessive levels (hyperglycemia) or not enough (hypoglycemia). Too much or too little blood glucose can lead to coma and even death if left untreated. This delicate balance becomes a challenge for all people with type 1 diabetes but can be effectively managed with appropriate treatment and self-care.

IN FOUR SEASONS as a softball second baseman for the University of California, Los Angeles, Kylee Perez batted .389, with 12 home runs and 98 RBIs (runs batted in). The Bruins advanced to the NCAA Women's College World Series in each of those seasons and, as a senior, Perez was named first-team All-Pac 12 and second-team All-American, starting all 65 of her team's games.

But years before Perez was a softball star at a powerhouse Division I program, she was an athletic dynamo in recreational leagues in her hometown of Alhambra, California.

By age 9, she played on basketball and softball teams. But soccer was her first love.

"I thought for sure I was going to grow up and be like Mia Hamm," Perez says, recalling her idol who led the University of North Carolina Tar Heels to four straight NCAA women's soccer titles.

After an otherwise ordinary soccer game, Perez's mother stood chatting with other soccer parents. Perez had worked up an appetite during the game and asked her mother if they could leave. But one conversation topic led to another, and the parents lingered as they packed up their soccer-watching gear.

"Mom! We need to leave!" she interrupted. "I need to eat, like, now!"

Today, Perez believes her insistence may have prevented a dangerous episode.

Perez's mom, Sonja, had noticed her daughter was eating more and frequently becoming ravenously hungry. But she also noticed her daughter was losing weight. It seemed normal for a growing, active, and energetic girl to get hungry a lot. But the weight loss was a worry. Sonja, a pediatric medical assistant, had a feeling something wasn't right with her daughter.

Perez also sensed something was off. At 9, she was long past the bedwetting stage. But a few nighttime accidents had her wondering what was going on.

Perez recalls a day in December 2006, at a pediatric appointment with her parents. After a blood test, she waited by herself while the doctor spoke with her parents.

"I sat there and, through the door, I could hear my mom crying," Perez recalls. "That's when I knew something was wrong."

After regaining her composure, Perez's mother came and got her.

"She told me, 'hey, you're going to be OK,'" Perez recalls. "'But we need to go the hospital right now.'"

Perez's diagnosis of diabetic ketoacidosis, a serious condition where high levels of acids build up in the blood because the body can no longer use glucose as an energy source, kept her in the hospital for a few days, as doctors did routine blood tests, replenished her fluids and electrolytes, and gave her insulin treatment. Her main fear, she says, wasn't the diabetes.

"I didn't even know what it was. I didn't cry because I had diabetes. I cried because I assumed I couldn't play sports."

The fears were short-lived. Perez's parents researched her disease and committed to doing everything possible to help their daughter lead whatever life she wanted to lead. However, the journey wasn't always smooth.

Signs and Symptoms of Newly Diagnosed Diabetes

- Classic symptoms of hyperglycemia (high blood glucose) can include frequent thirst, frequent urination, blurry vision, weight loss, and fatigue.

- At the time of diagnosis of any type of diabetes, the medical priorities include making sure dehydration and any electrolyte abnormalities are corrected. Depending on the severity of the disease, individuals may be treated in the outpatient or inpatient setting. Insulin therapy may be needed, particularly in type 1 diabetes or severe type 2 diabetes. The goal is to normalize electrolyte abnormalities, rehydrate, and bring glucose values down to a safer range.

- People with severe symptoms at the time of a type 1 diabetes diagnosis may present with diabetic ketoacidosis (DKA). This occurs when the body is not able to make any insulin. In response, the body uses fat as an energy source and produces blood ketones, which can lead to dangerous changes in the pH of the body. Untreated, this can lead to serious complications and possibly death. DKA is typically treated in an intensive care unit with intravenous insulin.

- The initial diagnosis of diabetes can be overwhelming for patients and family members. Education is critical for newly diagnosed patients. Priorities include learning how to take diabetes medications and inject insulin if needed, how to use a glucose meter to check blood glucose, how to treat a low blood glucose, and learning the effect of carbohydrates on blood glucose values.

"There was a lot of trial and error," says Perez. "Knowing what to bring to the field; packing insulin in an ice chest. There's so much that goes into it."

She credits her parents with teaching her that type 1 diabetes needn't limit her passion for athletic competition. "Whether it was buying the little carb-counting books, to my mom setting her alarm to go off in the middle of the night to wake up and test me."

Perez says that, after the initial tears of that first blood test, she and her family never looked back.

— Expert Commentary —

Diabetic ketoacidosis is a potentially life-threatening condition that can occur with type 1 diabetes, in particular, and requires immediate medical attention. It is commonly the presenting symptom when patients are first diagnosed with the disease. The signs and symptoms of newly diagnosed diabetes are shown in Box 1.1. Treatment includes intravenous hydration, insulin therapy, and correction of electrolytes in the hospital. With prompt care, diabetic ketoacidosis can be appropriately treated before serious complications occur.

Diabetic ketoacidosis rarely occurs in type 2 diabetes patients. These are typically patients with long-standing type 2 diabetes who have developed insulin deficiency (an inability to make insulin on their own) and require multiple injections of insulin daily. The treatment for diabetic ketoacidosis in these patients is similar to the treatment of type 1 diabetes patients with the same condition.

CATHY REESE knows all about late-night wakeups to test glucose. She also knows a little bit about coaching, having guided the University of Maryland Terrapins women's lacrosse team to five national championships.

Life as both head coach of the NCAA's premier women's lacrosse program and a mom of four means that, during the season, any combination of her children is likely to travel with her and the Terps to a game. On a long team bus ride to a game, Reese noticed her 7-year-old son Riley repeatedly visiting a cooler full of bottled water.

"He drank, like, three big bottles of water," she remembers. "I thought, jeez, how can a second-grader need that much water?"

A few other unusual symptoms sent Reese and Riley to the family's pediatrician for a checkup and a blood test a few days after the bus trip. When the physician called with news that her son has type 1 diabetes, Reese wasn't quite sure what it all meant.

"She told me to get Riley to a hospital," Reese recalls. "It was 10 o'clock at night when she called. I said, 'do we need to go right now?'"

The doctor responded that, if Riley were her own child, she'd take him right away.

During the two-day hospital stay to get Riley's glucose under control and to learn more about managing his condition, Reese says the hardest part was learning to give her little boy a shot.

"Oh, it was bad," Reese says. "'Don't do this to me, Mom!' Crying and screaming, all of it. He didn't understand. He was only 7."

Since even a coaching legend like Reese couldn't call a time-out on the lacrosse season, her Terps faced the University of Pennsylvania Quakers on the road the day Riley was discharged from the hospital. On the way to Philadelphia, the team bus made a stop at the hospital to pick up the head coach and her little boy.

Reese says that athletes and coaches are frequently good at compartmentalizing life events and crises in order to compete without distraction. But the ordeal that she and Riley had endured over the past few days was very much on the coach's mind when the Terps' bus pulled into the parking lot at Penn's legendary Franklin Field.

Reese and Quakers head coach Karen Corbett are old friends. As their teams warmed up for the game, the two coaches chatted at midfield. When Reese recounted her last few days and Riley's diagnosis, Corbett shared that she has a close relative with type 1 diabetes.

"She said it in such a normal way," says Reese, who learned that Corbett's relative leads an otherwise typical and healthy life. "That was the first time I thought, 'OK, maybe we can do this.'"

Still, with a high-pressure coaching job, a husband with his own coaching career, and a houseful of kids, including a 3-month-old, Reese says there were some long nights those first few weeks.

The early days of a diabetes diagnosis can be scary, both for the person with the diagnosis and for their caregivers. The pressure to get it right can feel overwhelming.

"You kind of live on a roller coaster, where every day is different," says Reese.

On top of his diabetes, Riley lives with celiac disease—another autoimmune disease, which prohibits him from eating foods that contain gluten, a protein found in certain grains, such as wheat.

"With celiac, the diabetes is more complicated from day to day. But no matter what, you manage. You make different decisions."

Riley wears an insulin pump and takes his own care seriously. He plays lacrosse and basketball, and he understands his body better all the time.

"At first, it was weird," Riley says. "I didn't understand it. And my friends didn't understand it. Now I just say, there's stuff I can't eat."

— *Expert Commentary* —

People with type 1 diabetes are also at risk for other autoimmune diseases, such as celiac disease. This occurs in about 6% of people with type 1 diabetes. Usually, celiac disease occurs after the diagnosis of type 1 diabetes, but sometimes it can happen the other way around. People with celiac disease are sensitive to the presence of gluten in their diet, such as wheat-containing breads or cereals. The presence of both type 1 diabetes and celiac disease may require more dietary changes, and meeting with a dietitian is especially helpful.

However, by avoiding gluten-containing foods, it can be managed although may be more complex, as well-described by Riley.

Because type 2 diabetes is not an autoimmune disease, the higher risk for conditions such as celiac disease, vitiligo, and other autoimmune processes is not present.

THE TYPE 1 DIABETES DIAGNOSIS hit 9-year-old Mark Andrews's physician father hard.

"My dad isn't a guy who shows a lot of emotion," says Andrews, a tight end with the NFL's Baltimore Ravens. "So, as a little kid, seeing tears rolling down his face at the doctor's office, I kind of knew then that this was going to change my life forever."

When Andrews couldn't get through a youth soccer game without needing two or three bathroom breaks, his father, a urologist, knew something wasn't right.

"Needing to stop over and over was a red flag," Andrews recalls. "My dad knew something was up."

He realizes now what an advantage he had to have a father who understood his disease.

"My dad is the reason I'm able to compete at a high level," says Andrews. "He helped me through learning the steps to take care of myself."

Andrews was named most valuable player of a soccer tournament his team played in only a few weeks after his diagnosis. That's when he realized diabetes wasn't going to stop him.

"My doctor wasn't thrilled that I was playing soccer again in the Arizona summer heat," Andrews says. "That's not really ideal for a kid with newly diagnosed type 1."

After a diabetes diagnosis, it's a good idea to learn how the disease affects your body. Taking things a little slowly is the right approach for many people. Conversely, people like Andrews charge right back into the fray and learn a different way. Every person experiences the disease differently.

By the time high school rolled around, Andrews's skills on the football field were obvious. In three seasons at wide receiver at Scottsdale, Arizona's Desert Mountain High School, Andrews caught 207 passes for 3,674 yards and 48 touchdowns. He also served as his team's punter and placekicker.

Andrews says his parents met with Desert Mountain's athletic trainers to ensure that they understood their son's condition.

"That was to make sure the trainers knew what to look for and what to do," Andrews says, in case he had a problem.

He says his diagnosis forced him into a certain self-reliance. "It's good to have a lot of eyes on you, whether that's your family or an athletic training staff. But I learned at an early age that, ultimately, you have to rely mostly on yourself."

Knowing his disease and its tendencies, understanding the signals his body is sending, and taking the appropriate action, says Andrews, remains his own responsibility.

"I think diabetes matured me a little faster," he says. "It meant things like, when friends or teammates might go and get a bunch of doughnuts, that's something I just wasn't going to be able to do. That's a luxury I just could never afford."

— Expert Commentary —

Mark Andrews was able to develop world-class athletic abilities despite his diagnosis of diabetes by learning to understand the disease and the impact on his training routine. Common presenting symptoms of any type of diabetes including the 3 Ps: polyuria (frequent urination), polydipsia (frequent thirst), and polyphagia (feeling hungry a lot). Blurry vision and unintentional weight loss are also common. When he required extra bathroom breaks during his soccer game, this was likely one of the first signs that his blood

---

BOX 1.2

How to Diagnose Diabetes

Diabetes is diagnosed by many different criteria:

- **Fasting blood test:** a blood glucose value of 126 md/dl or greater, after having nothing to eat or drink except water for at least 8–10 hours overnight.

- **Two-hour 75-gram oral glucose tolerance test:** a blood glucose value of 200 md/dl or greater, checked two hours after drinking a special sugary beverage containing 75 grams of carbohydrate as part of a glucose tolerance test. The individual needs to fast the night before the test.

- **Hemoglobin A1C test:** a blood hemoglobin A1C level 6.5% or greater. The A1C test gives an indication of average blood glucose values over the last 2–3 months and does not require the individual to be fasting.

- **Symptoms:** when someone has classic symptoms of high blood glucose with a random blood glucose value above 200 md/dl; usually this is confirmed with one of the tests above.

Only one positive test from the above criteria is needed for the diagnosis of diabetes. However, the diagnosis should be confirmed with a repeat blood test on a different day, or with another diagnostic test.

---

sugars were too high. In individuals who have symptoms of high blood glucose, blood tests should be conducted to confirm the diagnosis. The criteria used for diagnosis of diabetes are listed in Box 1.2.

A diabetes diagnosis shouldn't be taken lightly. It's a serious disease that requires attention. But it's not the end of the world. The best way to get off to a good start after a diabetes diagnosis is to find a supportive health care team that has experience with patients who have diabetes. Finding a good diabetes provider is the first step in that journey.

Diabetes doesn't have to mean the end of anything.

Chapter 2

Learning about Diabetes

Where did it come from?

A HIGH OR LOW BLOOD-SUGAR episode is never OK. But it's especially not OK at 225 miles per hour.

Well into his racing career when diagnosed at age 22, Charlie Kimball says he learns something new about his diabetes every time he climbs into a race car.

"Whether it was right after being diagnosed or the race just last weekend, I've learned something." His goal, he says, is "to make sure my diabetes becomes a nonfactor in my performance on the racetrack."

Because Indy race cars have so little room in them, the steering wheel serves as the car's dashboard. Right in front of the driver is a complicated display of gauges, buttons, dials, and digital readouts. The car's real-time data get transmitted wirelessly back to the driver's crew. Together, crew and driver keep a constant watch on telemetry, fuel maps, and switches to control hydraulics.

But Kimball's racing team outfitted his car with an extra sensor. Alongside displays of things like engine temperature, lap time, and tire pressure is a reading of Kimball's glucose. His continuous glucose monitor is integrated into his car's electronic data system, which sends information back to his pit crew.

His team's engineers also designed a special drink system for Kimball's car; when his glucose level looks like it might get low, Kimball drinks orange juice through a straw that snakes into his custom-made racing helmet. If he's just thirsty, a simple valve switch allows him to change from juice to water.

How much glucose he'll take in depends on where he is in the race.

"It's a different answer if I'm in lap one," he says, "than if I'm in lap 245 of a 248-lap race."

In Kimball's sport, behind the wheel of a car that travels 100 yards per second, a lapse in intense concentration could have consequences far more costly than just losing a position or two on the track.

"One of the things I think that separates great racing drivers from average drivers on the road is the ability to process information" at high speeds, he says. "You have to be looking and thinking a mile ahead."

At maximum speeds around 225 miles per hour, Kimball says he's "absorbing and processing a huge amount of data and information at all times, consciously and subconsciously. I'm deciding what's relevant and critical right now and then I'm filing away the rest." By now, he says, integrating his glucose numbers with the rest of the data "has almost become second nature."

He says it helps that he's not the only one paying attention to his glucose numbers. Just as his team monitors the car's tire pressure from the pit area, they also keep their eyes on his glucose levels.

"I don't come into Turn 1 at Indianapolis worried that the right front tire is flat because I know those guys are watching it," says Kimball. "Same goes for thinking about diabetes while I'm racing. The team is also watching my glucose values so I can concentrate on driving."

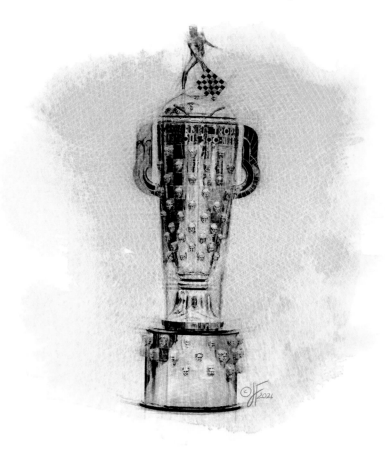

IndyCar trophy

— *Expert Commentary* —

Hypoglycemia is a major side effect of insulin therapy that can occur in people with diabetes and must be carefully monitored. Symptoms of hypoglycemia include feeling lightheaded, dizzy, sweaty, tremulous, or having heart palpitations. People with type 1 diabetes or type 2 diabetes who are on insulin therapy are more likely to experience hypoglycemia. People with type 2 diabetes on a class of medicines called sulfonylureas (glipizide, glimepiride, glyburide) are also at risk for hypoglycemia.

With severe hypoglycemia, the brain can be affected and coma is a serious concern. Low glucose levels are usually considered less than 70 mg/dl, and most people experience symptoms of hypoglycemia below this level. However, in people with type 1 diabetes who have episodes repeatedly, they may be unaware of deep drops in blood sugar since their bodies no longer trigger the appropriate warning signals called "hypoglycemia unawareness." In general, severe hypoglycemia can be dangerous and result in decreased concentration for high-performing athletes such as Charlie Kimball, which may ultimately impact his ability to compete if not treated right away. Self-monitoring of blood glucose levels and being aware of the symptoms of low blood glucose is key to preventing serious hypoglycemic events.

IN 2006, ADAM DRISCOLL, who was diagnosed at age 12 with type 1 diabetes, and his college buddies Patrick Blair and Jesse Stump decided to ride bicycles from Bellingham, Washington, to Ocean City, Maryland.

They'd raise money for diabetes research, as well as for a program to benefit kids with disabilities in African nations, another cause close to their hearts.

Under any circumstances, riding bikes from one end of the United States to the other is a monumental undertaking. But Driscoll and his pals added three elements to their journey that made it even more unusual.

The first element was the path they decided to follow.

If any bicycle route from the northwest tip of the continental United States to a resort town on the Atlantic Ocean can be called typical, then the typical route would take riders a little more than 3,100 miles through 13 states. They would stretch across the northernmost slice of the country, through Idaho, Montana, the Dakotas, past the Great Lakes, and into Pennsylvania to the eastern shore of Maryland.

But Driscoll's gang decided instead to avoid the steepest mountains on the trip. The Rockies and the Appalachians present some awfully tough climbs for even the most seasoned cyclists riding high-tech, multispeed bikes.

But the second unusual element helped with their decision to ride south as they made their way east.

That element: fixed-gear bicycles.

When you learned to ride a bicycle, chances are its chain was looped over a single sprocket. Later, maybe you got a 3-speed or even a 10- or 12-speed bike that allowed you to take hills more easily.

But "fixies," as they're known, have only one speed. That speed? Whatever speed your legs can generate. Uphill, downhill, and flat surfaces all use the same gear. Many bike messengers and other urban cyclists ride fixed-gear bikes for their efficiency in transferring the rider's energy from the pedal to the drivetrain. One pedal equals one turn of the wheels.

But for long road journeys, like the one Driscoll and his buddies were undertaking, multispeed bikes are much more the norm.

Driscoll says they encountered more than a few doubters when they began seeking support for their fixed-gear adventure. Plenty of cyclists ride across the country. But very few do it without some help from the gears on the bikes.

"A lot of people told us we were nuts," he laughs. "They thought we'd ruin our knees or something. But we wanted to do something that would stand out. None of us had even been riding fixies for very long. We just really liked the idea."

The final unusual element of the gang's journey was a decision they made early on, before they left the state of Washington. They decided they needed to sing karaoke in every state through which they rode.

Why karaoke? Driscoll still laughs when he answers.

"Because who *does* that?"

BOX 2.1

Understanding How Carbohydrates Get Digested

At halftime of your recreation league soccer game, you're feeling pretty good—but maybe a little tired. You've spent 45 minutes running hard, playing both offense and defense. Your muscles are warm and loose, your heart is pumping oxygenated blood to every part of your body, and you've got a healthy sweat going. You've used your brain to make split-second decisions on whether to pass or shoot, whether to tackle or defend. Your face is flushed, and your breathing is heavier than normal. The exertion has made you thirsty and you don't quite have the fresh legs you had at kickoff.

On the sidelines, while your coach encourages your team and adjusts strategies for the second half, you dig into your equipment bag and pull out a big bottle of water and a banana.

The water will hydrate your muscles and joints, refresh your body's trillions of cells, and help maintain your normal body temperature, even while you're hustling on the pitch. And under that banana's yellow peel is the fuel that will propel your body through the second half.

But how? It's just a banana. What makes it a source of energy?

In addition to replacing the vitamins and minerals you've spent during warmups and the first half, that banana will top off your energy tank with about 25–30 grams of carbohydrates. The carbohydrate composition of bananas changes drastically during ripening. Unripe bananas contain resistant starch, a type of carbohydrate that "resists" digestion in the small intestine. It is absorbed slowly and does not cause sharp rises in blood sugar. As bananas ripen, the starch is converted to sugars. The most common types of sugar in ripe bananas are sucrose, fructose, and glucose. Bananas have a relatively low glycemic index, a measurement of how quickly carbs in food enter your bloodstream and raise blood sugar, depending on their ripeness. All these attributes make them an ideal halftime energy boost.

You eat the banana and, almost immediately, your body's fuel system snaps into action. After the banana hits your stomach and the rest of your gut, a slurry of enzymes will break down the fruit into its most basic elements. The banana's carbohydrates become special types of sugars that will boost your body's fuel supply for the second half.

Just beneath the liver, tucked between every person's stomach and spine is a pancreas—a flat, 6-inch organ that drives how our bodies convert food into nutrition.

Part of the pancreas's job is to produce insulin from clusters of cells scattered throughout the pancreas called "islets." Insulin is a hormone that tells the body's cells—primarily in the muscle, fat, and liver—to absorb the sugars that, just a few minutes ago, were housed in your banana. When the cells receive the signal from the insulin, they open their doors to absorb just the right amount of sugars to keep your glucose levels in the target range and your whole system balanced and energized while you sprint, kick, block, and tackle through the second half.

But what happens if your body's cells don't get the message the insulin is sending? Or what if your pancreas can't produce insulin? If your body can't adequately respond to the message the insulin is sending, it responds by sending a stronger signal—or more insulin. This is called "insulin resistance" and is central to the development of type 2 diabetes.

On the other hand, if your body can't produce insulin at all due to proteins (called auto-antibodies) that mistake the pancreas as foreign and "self-attack" the body, then the insulin-producing islets in the pancreas shut down and type 1 diabetes develops.

Without the action of insulin, the body cannot lower blood glucose levels, leading to many short- and long-term complications if left untreated.

— *Expert Commentary* —

Planning ahead for prolonged periods of physical activity is critically important when you have diabetes. In particular, having plenty of carbohydrate sources on board and eating regularly is key to keep blood glucose levels in check. Understanding carbohydrate digestion is complex (Box 2.1) but a matter of survival when you have type 1 diabetes. Planning may also be

necessary for people with type 2 diabetes, especially in those treated with insu-
lin or sulfonylureas. Exercise in combination with these medicines can lead to
hypoglycemia, so planning for sources of carbohydrates is important.

BY THE TIME LAUREN COX entered her senior season at Baylor University, the 6-foot, 4-inch forward had won pretty much all there was to win in the world of women's amateur college basketball.

She came to Baylor as the nation's top-rated prospect at her position, after leading Flower Mound (Texas) High School to four straight district championships. Playing in the Big 12, one of America's most competitive conferences for women's basketball, Cox won a national championship in 2019 and was named Player of the Year in 2020.

Cox has always been athletic. She says that, as a child, she "played a little bit of everything—soccer, basketball, volleyball. I was running track too."

Diagnosed with type 1 diabetes at age 7, Cox says her hometown endocrinologist was instrumental in keeping her in the games.

"She was always really encouraging," says Cox. "We worked together and tried new things. She was always there to help me out."

Adjusting basal rates of her insulin pump throughout the day, she says, was a frequent topic.

"Every time I'd go to see her, we would tweak things to try to make them just a little better," Cox says. For example, "Like, my sugar would always go high after I ate breakfast. So, we increased my basal [rate] in the morning, just to keep it in a good range through the day."

While Cox is comfortable managing her diabetes, it hasn't always been easy.

"There were days when I just broke down because it was so difficult," she admits. "Some days, your sugar might be high and you don't know what's going on. You've changed your [insulin pump supplies] set and you've changed your insulin and your blood sugar is still high. It's so frustrating and you just don't know what else to do."

Cox comes from a family steeped in Texas basketball. The oldest of four girls, Cox's parents both played in college, her father Dennis at Central Methodist University and her mother Brenda at Southern Methodist University. Her sister Whitney, who plays at NCAA Division II Lubbock Christian, was diagnosed with type 1 diabetes at age 17, while Cox was at Baylor.

Over her years of athletic competition, Cox has never had a teammate with diabetes. In fact, none of her coaches had ever coached a player who had the disease. Throughout her basketball career, Cox's parents have instructed her coaches on managing their daughter's diabetes.

"I was really close with my high school and AAU [Amateur Athletic Union] coaches," she says. "They were both really open to learning what they could do. And of course, I had my parents there too."

By her senior season at Flower Mound, Cox was among the most heavily recruited high school players in the nation. Powerhouse women's basketball schools all wanted a player with the size and versatility Cox offered. She visited five big-time NCAA programs before deciding on nearby Baylor as the school for her.

During each visit, Cox's diabetes was a topic of discussion. Dennis, Brenda, and Lauren grilled team trainers and doctors, in addition to coaching staffs.

When the time came to talk with head coaches, Cox says her mother asked each one the same question: "If y'all are playing in the national championship game and Lauren has high or low blood sugar, what are you doing to do?"

It was the ultimate question. If, in the biggest game a coach, a team, and a university athletic program could play, would the coach make the decision to favor a player's health and safety over a national title?

Cox recalls that Baylor head coach Kim Mulkey's answer to the question was simple.

"She said, 'Lauren's not playing.' That was pretty much it."

Cox spent her freshman season learning the ropes of big-time college basketball, averaging 7.6 points and almost one and a half blocked shots per game on her way to the Big 12 All-Freshman Team. The next season, as a starter, she doubled those numbers and added nearly 10 rebounds per game. The Bears went 33–2 for the season, winning the Big 12 regular season and tournament before being upset in the NCAA quarterfinals by Oregon State.

Cox's junior season was the one Bears fans will remember for a long time. Top-ranked Baylor's 37–1 record took them all the way to the national championship game against third-ranked Notre Dame.

Coach Mulkey did have to remove Cox from the game late in the third quarter. But it wasn't diabetes that sent her to the locker room. It was her knee.

With 1:22 remaining in the quarter, the Bears led the Fighting Irish by 12 points. Cox was on her way to a great personal performance (8 points and 8 rebounds) and a national championship when, in a loose-ball scrum under the Irish basket, she got tangled up with a teammate and her left knee bent in the wrong direction. Immediately, Cox crumpled to the floor and, after several minutes of on-court medical attention from trainers, was helped to the locker room. Her national championship night ended with eight points, eight rebounds, and three blocked shots.

Without its star player, Baylor watched its 17-point lead evaporate in the game's waning minutes. The Bears barely survived Notre Dame's furious surge and hung on for an 82–81 win, the university's third-ever women's basketball national title. Mulkey called Cox "the heart and soul" of the national championship team.

While serious, Cox's injury looked a lot worse than it was. During the fourth quarter, she returned to her team's bench on crutches to thunderous cheers from Baylor supporters among the 20,000 fans in Tampa's Amalie Arena. Cox was able to take part in the on-court victory celebration with her teammates.

After two months of rehabilitation and physical therapy to heal and strengthen her knee, Cox was ready for her senior season. She missed a handful of games in late 2019 to a foot injury but was named Big 12 Player of the Year at season's end.

For their determination and their advocacy for kids with diabetes, Cox and her younger sister Whitney were co-winners of the Pat Summitt Most Courageous Award, an NCAA honor named for the legendary University of Tennessee women's basketball coach whose life and coaching career were cut short by early-onset Alzheimer's disease.

The Big 12 and NCAA tournaments were canceled in 2020 due to the COVID-19 pandemic. But Cox made her mark during the regular season, showing pro scouts that not only was she fully recovered from the knee injury but that her game had improved: a shot blocker who can shoot 3-pointers and a scorer who also dishes out assists. The WNBA predraft scouting report told the story; there were players in the draft who averaged more points, rebounds, assists, steals, and blocks than Lauren Cox. But only Cox possessed a combination of each of those skills.

On 2020 WNBA draft night, Cox was the third player selected, the first-round pick of the Indiana Fever. After two seasons which featured various injuries and a COVID-19 diagnosis, Cox signed a mid-season contract with the Los Angeles Sparks in June 2021.

— *Expert Commentary* —

Cox candidly shares how some days living with diabetes can be more difficult than others. Though competitive athletes may at times seem to have superhuman abilities, they can also feel overwhelmed or angry just like anyone else. With a chronic disease, it is not uncommon to have feelings of frustration or to be discouraged at times. Diabetes is a disease that relies heavily on the ability

BOX 2.2

What's the Difference between Type 1 and Type 2 Diabetes?

What is type 1 diabetes?

Your body's immune system, which, under most circumstances, is very good at fending off things like harmful viruses and bacteria that can cause illness, kills the special cells in your own pancreas that produce insulin.

Antibodies are proteins produced in the blood that are weapons against bacteria, viruses, and other contagions that the body recognizes as harmful. When we're exposed to the virus that causes the common cold, for instance, a battle erupts inside our bodies. Antibodies fight back the invaders, working hard to prevent them from replicating and taking hold. During these epic struggles that take place inside our bodies, we might feel a little run-down or sniffly, but mainly, we're able to go about our regular business. From time to time, the viruses take the lead, leaving us feeling lousy for a few days while the antibodies catch up and finally win the day.

But autoimmune diseases cause the body to produce antibodies that fight against its own systems. The body mistakenly believes it's under attack when it's not. Conditions like lupus, Crohn's disease, and even psoriasis are the results of very specific malfunctions of the immune system.

Type 1 diabetes, sometimes known as juvenile diabetes or insulin-dependent diabetes, is also an autoimmune disease that scientists and researchers believe is usually caused by a defective gene but that can also be triggered by exposure to certain viruses. Though the last few decades have seen enormous strides in understanding and treating type 1 diabetes, there still is no cure for the disease.

If you have type 1 diabetes, your body's immune system attacked and destroyed the cells in your pancreas that produced insulin. It can occur at any age, and also in adulthood, but the most common ages are in childhood between 4 and 7 years, then again between 10 and 14 years.

What is type 2 diabetes?

Type 2 diabetes is a little different. The pancreas makes insulin, but the body's cells no longer respond to it. Insulin resistance typically comes from a number of factors. First, there's usually a family history component to it. Having a first-degree relative with type 2 diabetes, such as a parent or sibling, increases risk substantially. Also, certain races and ethnicities are more likely than others to develop type 2 diabetes.

People of Asian, Hispanic, and African descent are at greater type 2 diabetes risk than people whose descendants were European. Still, ethnicity is only one factor in diabetes risk and there are likely multiple genetic factors. Smoking is also a risk factor.

Body weight plays an important role in how your cells respond to insulin, and excess body fat makes your body more resistant to the effects of insulin. Being overweight can lead to type 2 diabetes, especially as you age. One of the reasons that, over the past few decades, the United States has seen type 2 diabetes rise to epidemic levels are diets that have grown higher in refined sugars and carbohydrates. Not coincidentally, an estimated two-thirds of Americans are considered overweight or obese.

If type 2 diabetes is not treated or doesn't improve, the insulin resistance process can take a toll on the pancreas and lead to burnout or death of insulin-producing cells in the islets and a state of insulin deficiency.

Type 2 diabetes usually occurs in adulthood. However, children with obesity, especially those from minority racial or ethnic groups, are more prone to developing it.

of the patient to self-manage their disease at home, including both type 1 and type 2 diabetes (Box 2.2). This can take time to learn and having the support of family, teammates, and coaches can be a tremendous boost for an individual with diabetes.

KYLEE PEREZ has relied on insulin pumps since the fifth grade.

"Before that, I was using needles. But I'm in love with the technology," she says, referring to the tools that are available to help her manage diabetes now.

The softball player uses a continuous glucose monitor (CGM), an insulin pump, and her knowledge of her own body to keep her type 1 diabetes under control.

"I know not everyone with diabetes can recognize their own highs and lows," she says, "but luckily for me, I can. I can feel it when things aren't quite right."

Many athletes with diabetes eat the same food and exercise the same way on practice days and follow similar routines on game days, based on what time their competition will take place. Perez says she doesn't follow a routine as strict as many other athletes.

"I know I can eat the exact same thing every day and my sugar still can be different every day," she says. "I pay attention to my body and to my CGM. I just kind of live it day by day."

On days when things aren't working right or her sugar is hard to control, Perez says it's important to resist getting discouraged.

"No matter what, there are no failures. I can have a day where I do everything perfectly and I still have zero control over what's going on," she says. "I heard someone say something that I try to live my entire life by: 'It's never a failure; it's always a lesson.'"

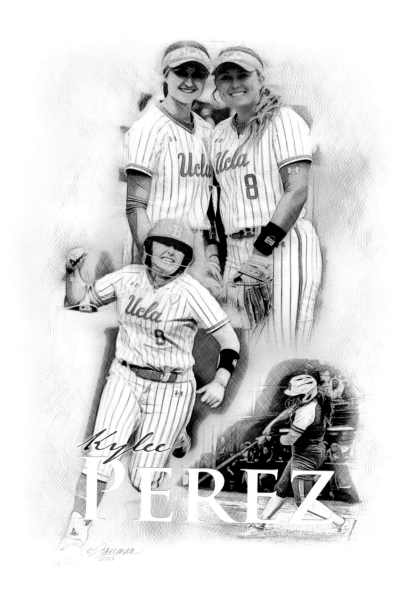

Kylee Perez, American softball player who played for
the University of California, Los Angeles, four-time All-Pac-12 player:
"It's never a failure; it's always a lesson."

— Expert Commentary —

The insulin pump is a handheld device that delivers insulin continuously, usually through a catheter placed under the skin. This is an alternative to multiple daily injections of insulin and is often used in people with type 1 diabetes. It helps many patients to maintain glucose levels in the target range, both between and during meals, while improving quality of life.

DOUG BURNS was 42 years old when he was crowned Natural Mr. Universe, the highest drug-tested achievement a bodybuilder can attain.

But as a child, Burns was alarmingly small. At age 12, he weighed only 53 pounds, far short of normal weight for his age.

His story reads like the old advertisement in the back of comic books, where the beach bully kicks sand in the skinny kid's face. Diagnosed with type 1 diabetes at age 7, Burns spent his early school years living with his parents outside Washington, DC, the target of merciless abuse from other kids.

"I was the smallest kid in my class. Boys, girls, it didn't matter. They all picked on me," he remembers. "It was like the school sport."

During Burns's early-1970s childhood, treatment for diabetes was still primitive. Human insulin would not be available for another decade; animals were the only source. Diabetes monitoring and care was, at best, inexact.

Glucose tests were performed by adding urine to a bottle with a blue substance known as Benedict's solution. The sample was heated on a stove for several minutes and changed colors to indicate whether the patient's sugar was high. There was no test for low blood glucose at the time; if a person began feeling the symptoms of low

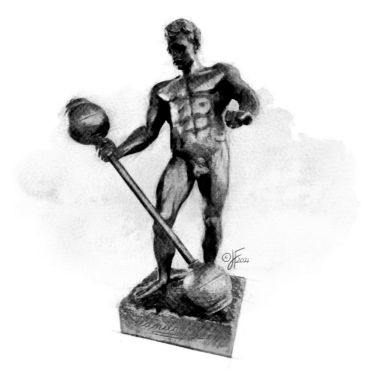

Mr. Olympia bodybuilding championship trophy

blood sugar, he or she just ate or drank something with sugar in it. Orange juice or candy would launch blood sugar back up. How high would it go? No one knew.

Burns believes now that, while his parents took him to many of the nation's top hospitals to work with pediatric diabetes specialists, they didn't understand the disease well and were less diligent about its management than they could have been. His father was a space scientist and the Burns family was largely consumed by his work.

His mismanaged diabetes was affecting his growth. Years later, Burns would realize why he nearly always felt sick and had such trouble gaining weight.

"I was in ketoacidosis. I was emaciated and dehydrated."

Burns is at pains to explain the logic, but despite his ill health, neither he nor his parents took diabetes especially seriously.

He spent more of his fifth-grade year in hospitals than in school. During one hospital stay, Burns recalls, a doctor who was familiar with his case told him he wanted to introduce him to someone.

The doctor brought the 11-year-old boy to a dialysis center in the hospital and introduced him to a man who was undergoing the procedure that helps patients whose kidneys no longer function to clear their bodies of waste, salt, and fluid, as well as replenish the supply of important minerals and electrolytes.

"The man getting dialysis was decrepit," Burns remembers. "His whole system was just coming apart."

Seated next to a loud, bulky dialysis machine, the man was undergoing the procedure that cleans toxins from the blood when kidneys no longer function. Over the course of about half a day, the man's blood would pump through a large needle in his arm and then through a long tube into the machine that filtered out waste. As blood was cleaned, it was returned back to the man through another needle and long tube. The process also replaced important nutrients that his body could no longer retain on its own.

While the dialysis machine hummed, the man recounted to Burns his years of inattention to his diabetes and the life-threatening health complications he endured as a result. His implication was clear: this is where you're headed.

Walking back toward Burns's hospital room, the physician asked the boy one last question.

"Now do you understand how serious this disease is?"

A young Doug Burns knew diabetes was bad, but "I figured these guys were trying to scare me," he says now.

The look on his face must've given away his skepticism. Burns says what happened next changed his life.

"The doctor stopped walking, looked right at me, put his hands up and said, 'suit yourself.' And he left me standing right there."

The 11-year-old, who was 30 pounds underweight, watched his doctor walk down a long hospital corridor.

"I didn't know where to go or what to do," Burns says. "I just stood there crying."

The wisdom of a medical professional frightening and abandoning a young child is debatable. But Burns says the moment transformed the way he thought about diabetes and his own health.

"It was hard, but I needed that doctor's message desperately. From that point forward, I tried to get my sugars under control myself. And I finally started gaining a little weight."

— Expert Commentary —

Long-term complications of any type of diabetes include eye disease (retinopathy), nerve damage (neuropathy), kidney failure (nephropathy), heart disease, and stroke and can occur with any type of diabetes. However, if blood glucose levels are optimally managed, this can dramatically delay the progression or prevent onset of complications. More than half of patients with end-stage kidney disease on dialysis has diabetes. Modification of cardiovascular risk factors such as blood pressure and cholesterol management, smoking cessation, and preventive therapy with aspirin or cholesterol drugs when appropriate is also important to prevent complications.

It's easy to imagine that racing is the oldest form of competition. The fundamental simplicity of testing who can be the first to arrive at Point B from Point A is surely as old as the concept of competition itself.

Any kind of race—swimming, running, driving, cycling—requires contestants to push hard enough to finish before the other competitors. Maybe maximum effort isn't necessary. Maybe conditioning and strategy are enough to propel a contestant over the line sooner than a superior athlete.

At low levels of competition, racers' abilities tend to have wide gaps. In races like high school track meets or Saturday night dirt-track oval driving, the finishes are as likely as not to be lopsided. A slow start. A wide turn. A stumble. Each costs valuable time and distance. The winner will be the contestant who makes the fewest errors and is best able to recover from them.

At elite levels of racing, though, the variance in skill levels among athletes is minimal. Mistakes are far less common. If the difference between first and second place is measured in milliseconds, athletes seek every possible advantage they can find, no matter how small. These include swimming caps and hairless bodies, wind-drag reduction systems on race cars, and bicycles that weigh barely 15 pounds.

When Olympic swimmer Gary Hall Jr. decided he wanted to continue competing against the fastest swimmers in the world, he knew he was starting every race at a disadvantage: no one else in the pool would have diabetes.

After his diagnosis, Hall continued training for the 2000 Olympic Games, which were less than 18 months away. He stayed with his routine, switching between his hometown of Phoenix and his team's training center in Berkeley, California. He chugged sports drinks between practice swims; his blood sugar plummeted and spiked daily—it was a constant fight between the hypoglycemia brought on by the intensity of his grueling workouts and the sharp increase in blood sugar that comes from sucking down a quart of Powerade in a few giant gulps.

Hall compares training for the Olympics to learning about diabetes. Both require "consistency and hard work," he says. Swimming laps and perfecting techniques are akin, says Hall, to finger sticks and insulin injections. "Finding out what works best, trying new things, making adjustments—they're all part of learning."

Given his diagnosis experience, which amounted to a short lesson in giving himself insulin shots, Hall needed to find a doctor who specialized in diabetes and athletic competition. Hall knew that, if he were to continue competing—and winning—against the best swimmers in the world, he would need "near-perfect diabetes management and a near-perfect swim."

He heard about an endocrinologist in Los Angeles who had worked with other athletes and decided to make an appointment.

"The plan was to fly to LA, meet the doctor, and fly back home," Hall recalls. "But naturally, my flight was delayed and I got to her office just as she was leaving."

On her way out the door, she told Hall she was driving across town to give a talk. He was welcome to join her on the drive, she said. The two could talk and see if she was the right fit to help him stay at the top levels of competitive swimming. No guarantees, no commitments. Just fact finding.

The 6-foot, 6-inch Hall folded himself into the physician's Volkswagen Beetle and the pair began the trek across LA. Zooming down the Santa Monica Freeway, the endocrinologist asked Hall specific questions about his training regimen, his condition, and his experience so far with diabetes. By the time they reached the physician's speaking engagement, she agreed to be his diabetes doctor.

"She didn't make any promises about how well I would do or even whether it could work," Hall says. "She told me nobody had ever done it before, but that, 'sure, let's give it a try.'"

"For me, it was a giant relief—the best thing that could've happened."

At the Sydney Games, Hall became the first US athlete to compete in the Olympics with type 1 diabetes. By the time the Games ended, Hall would become the only Olympic swimmer with diabetes ever to earn a medal, taking home four. He won the gold medal for 50-meter individual freestyle, a bronze in the 100-meter freestyle, and a gold and silver in team relays. Four years later, in the Games at Athens, at age 29, Hall was oldest American swimmer to compete in 80 years. He won the 50-meter freestyle gold medal again, as well as a bronze in the 4 × 100-meter freestyle relay.

— *Expert Commentary* —

Gary Hall Jr. shares how the ups and downs of blood glucose levels that commonly occurred during his training were an additional challenge that he had to overcome in order to be successful at his sport. However, fluctuations in blood glucose levels are a daily challenge for all people with diabetes. Understanding patterns, particularly how the body responds to different types of physical activity and recommendations for dietary intake (Box 2.3), is important.

Historically, urine test strips were used to measure home glucose levels but were not able to give numerical results—only whether readings were high. There is now a plethora of home blood glucose meters available to measure blood glucose using a pinprick of the finger. Patients on multiple daily injections of insulin or insulin pumps often require testing their blood glucose four or more times per day. In particular, athletes may need to check more frequently during rigorous activity to guard against blood sugars going too high or too low.

One of the keys to succeeding in athletics is being able to adapt when conditions change. When football fields get muddy, the players wear

BOX 2.3
Dietary Recommendations in Diabetes

Diabetes affects different people different ways. Thus, dietary recommendations depend on a person's age, other conditions the person lives with, and the amount of physical activity the person gets.

For people with type 1 diabetes, most of the focus is on carbohydrates. Knowing how many and the type of carbohydrates you're about to consume in a meal can help prevent large increases in blood glucose after the meal. Diabetes care providers often work with their type 1 patients to find an ideal ratio of insulin to carbohydrates. For instance, one unit of insulin for every 10 grams of carbohydrates. People with type 1 diabetes need to become familiar with counting the carbohydrates on their plate, then using the recommended ratio to help come to a before-meal insulin dose. Too much insulin can cause a low glucose episode after the meal. And too little can trigger a high glucose event.

Not all carbohydrates are created equal. Refined and processed sugars, also known as simple carbohydrates, are absorbed quickly and will raise glucose values rapidly. Complex carbohydrates are high in fiber and usually take much longer to digest and raise glucose values more slowly. For example, let's compare a glass of apple juice to a plate of vegetables. The two might have similar carbohydrate numbers, but that's where the similarities end. The juice is comprised of simple sugars that are easier to digest and will raise blood glucose levels more rapidly than the vegetables.

Physical activity plays an important role here. Exercise burns glucose and makes muscles more sensitive to insulin. A patient may find that 1 unit for 10 grams of carbohydrates is a good dose on a typical day. But let's say today is a rainy Sunday in October and you lay on the couch all day watching football. You might find that your body is less sensitive to the effects of insulin.

The following Sunday, however, is beautiful. Crisp, cool fall weather makes you want to play some touch football. You and your friends play hard until the sun begins to set. On a day like this, you might find that your body is more sensitive to the effects of insulin and that you only need 1 unit of insulin for 15 grams of carbohydrates during vigorous physical activity.

For type 2 diabetes, the dietary recommendations vary widely again based on the individual. But in general, some basic concepts apply. Weight loss is key for type 2 diabetes. Reducing weight reduces the burden of insulin resistance. Eating fewer calories than the caloric expenditure with activity is crucial for weight loss. Eating a moderate amount—not eliminating but limiting—of carbohydrates helps reduce large boosts of glucose after meals. In general, aiming for a healthy body mass index (usually <25 kg/m² for most individuals) or a goal of a 5% weight loss (for a 200-pound person, that would be a goal of a 10-pound weight loss) is recommended.

The US Centers for Disease Control and Prevention (CDC) and American Diabetes Association (ADA) both recommend the diabetes plate method; this includes filling about half your 9-inch dinner plate with non-starchy vegetables, such as salad, green beans, broccoli, cauliflower, cabbage, and carrots; fill one-quarter with a lean protein, such as chicken, turkey, beans, tofu, or eggs; and fill a quarter with a grain or starchy food, such as potatoes, rice, or pasta (or skip the starch altogether and double up on non-starchy veggies). If type 2 diabetes progresses to a point where insulin therapy is required, similar concepts of carbohydrate counting that are described above for type 1 diabetes above are often followed.

shoes with longer cleats. When a baseball manager brings in a left-handed relief pitcher, the opposing manager will frequently counter with a right-handed pinch hitter.

The athletes in this chapter all made adjustments to their routines and their lives so that they could continue competing in the sports they love. The same drive and determination that pushes them to excel in sports pushes them to make diabetes a nonfactor.

Chapter 3

Living with Diabetes
How will I manage day-to-day?

EVEN AS A CHILD, Jason Johnson was athletic. When he was diagnosed at 11 with type 1 diabetes, he wondered if it meant he could no longer play sports.

Both his doctor and his parents told him he could do whatever he wanted, as long as he paid attention to his diabetes. Johnson has given that same advice to the hundreds of kids with type 1 diabetes he has tried to inspire.

"I tell them that it's not the end of the world," he explains. "Don't let this be the end of you. Use it as a building block to make you a better person and a stronger person."

Having diabetes, he says, just means "you have to try a little harder than everybody else."

As a 20-year-old minor-league pitcher in Augusta, Georgia, five seasons before he would first pitch in the majors for the Pittsburgh Pirates, Johnson earned just barely enough money to make sure he had food in the house.

"There were four of us players living together, so we could afford the rent," he recalls. The teammates pooled their grocery money, "so

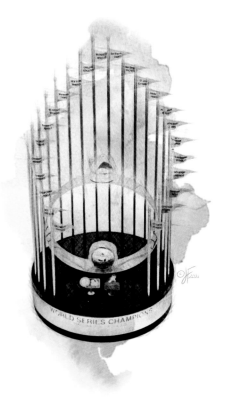

Major League Baseball World Series championship trophy

we could buy, like, normal food." But because Johnson has type 1 diabetes, he needed to make sure he had food that could help him when his blood sugar got low.

"I was always completely out of money by the end of the month," Johnson laughs.

He says that each year, as he moved through the minors to the major leagues, he learned more about pitching—and more about pitching with diabetes.

"By the time I got to the double-A level" in 1997, he says, "I pretty much had the day-to-day basics down. And it's a good thing, too. Because I got called up to the big leagues that same season. If I hadn't worked out a good system [to manage diabetes], who knows how that would've gone. In baseball, there are always players right behind you ready to take your spot. If I messed anything up with my blood sugars or my diabetes, the Pirates could always just call somebody else up and send me back down to the minors."

So, what was Johnson's magical nutrition secret? It's probably not what any physician would recommend, but Johnson swears that eating two McDonald's cheeseburgers helped his pitching.

"It started in the minors," he laughs. "Then in the majors, I stayed with it. A lot of times, there wouldn't be a McDonald's anywhere near our team hotel. So, I'd get in a cab and ride all over the place to get my cheeseburgers."

Johnson says now that his game-day cheeseburger routine had more to do with superstition than with good nutrition.

"Baseball players are the most superstitious people out there," says Johnson. "It became a superstition that I couldn't drop."

— *Expert Commentary* —

Two cheeseburgers from McDonald's? Not your typical athlete's pre-competition meal and not one many health care providers would recommend. But why might this have worked well for Jason Johnson? Carbohydrates alone are not the whole story when blood sugars rise. Simple carbohydrates (sugars found in cookies, candy, and juices) will quickly raise blood sugars. More complex carbohydrates (like brown rice, wheat bread, and broccoli) raise blood sugars more slowly.

Fat plays a big role too. A cheeseburger has carbohydrates but has plenty of fat as well—the cheese and the beef patty both have a large fat content. Fat in foods increases insulin resistance and make injections of insulin work less efficiently. In addition, the fat slows intestinal motility, which means it slows down the overall absorption of a meal by the gut, which then dampens the rise of blood sugars. The fiber and protein content also helps slow carbohydrate absorption and stabilizes blood sugar by slowing the release of glucose into the bloodstream. Consequently, foods such as a cheeseburger, pizza, or burrito have a more sustained and delayed rise in blood sugars after ingestion.

Johnson may have found his cheeseburgers so effective because they gave him a sustained rise in blood sugars over a few hours that prevented him from getting low blood sugars when he was on the mound.

AT 10 YEARS OLD, Kate Hall-Harnden experienced two events that would change her life forever: one, she was diagnosed with type 1 diabetes, and two, she discovered track and field.

Hall-Harnden currently holds the US outdoor high school long jump record, which she broke as a senior in 2015 with a jump of 22 and a half feet. That record had stood for 39 years and was set by a jumper who later won an Olympic silver medal.

Hall-Harnden had her sights on an Olympic medal of her own. She was training for a spot on the US team that would compete in the 2020 games in Tokyo when she hyperextended her left knee.

"Initially, I was confident it was just sore from the hyperextension," Hall-Harnden wrote in an Instagram post to announce the news. "But after an MRI, I found out that I completely tore my ACL."

As she healed from surgery to repair her anterior cruciate ligament, Hall-Harnden served as an assistant track coach at Saint Joseph's College near Portland, Maine. She also started a foundation called DiaStrong, which aims to help people with diabetes get healthy through exercise.

Hall-Harnden has always followed her own path, whether in athletics or in managing her diabetes. Like many elite American track athletes, she attended college on an athletic scholarship. Universities provide coaching, conditioning facilities, equipment, and everything else a track athlete needs to compete at the highest levels of the sport.

After her freshman season at Iowa State University, Hall-Harnden transferred to the University of Georgia, where she won national championships in the 60-meter sprint as well as the long jump.

Hall-Harnden says that, while she loved her teammates at Georgia, she felt the one-size-fits-all conditioning approach that is common in the NCAA was an impediment to her goal of jumping in the Olympics.

"I didn't like the NCAA system and how the coaches treated athletes," she says. "I wanted to focus on my own career and making the Olympic team. That's my ultimate goal."

Hall-Harnden was homeschooled as a high school student, a factor she credits as important to her ability to figure things out for herself. She made the decision to leave the University of Georgia after her junior season, returning to her quiet New England hometown to train with her high school coach.

"I've been independent since I was really young," she says. "And I was very motivated. I planned every day on my own. I didn't have to be in school all day, then practice at the end of a long day."

Hall-Harnden believes her ability to adjust her own training regimen set her on the path that led to her long jump record. But her college coaches insisted on a more general, less customized approach.

"Because I have diabetes, I need more recovery time" than other track athletes, she says. At Georgia, "our team workouts were extremely hard and we were practicing three or four hours a day, lifting really heavy weights."

Twenty-four hours after a grueling workout, Hall-Harnden's teammates could be ready to do it all over again.

"There were a lot of times where I was training at 70 or 80%," she says, "and my teammates were at 100%, just because their bodies were able to recover faster."

She says that college athletics clashed with her independence.

"It felt like I was being treated like a kid," she says of her college years. "If I wasn't having a good day in practice, the coaches assumed I was slacking off. I wasn't. I was sore. I needed to recover."

While Hall-Harnden's workouts are rigorous, they're customized to her own body and her own system.

Hall-Harnden has experimented with different insulin-delivery systems during her track and field career. She has settled on an Omnipod, a tubeless insulin pump a bit bigger than the size of a half dollar that Hall-Harnden affixes to the back of one of her upper arms. Along with a continuous glucose monitor, which she attaches to her abdomen, this pump device helps her to adjust her insulin doses so that her glucose levels are in a good range during practice and competition.

In high school, Hall-Harnden says, she was frustrated by bulky insulin pumps with long tubes attached.

"I had to disconnect the pump for the whole competition," she says, explaining the difficulty of sprinting or jumping with an insulin pump. "And back then, I was doing three or four different events in a meet. So, I would run from event to event with no insulin. By the time I was done, I'd leave the meet with ketones."

Hall-Harnden says she considered giving up on track and field as a result of her trouble with insulin pumps.

"I was really discouraged," she recalls. "It's the only time I've felt that diabetes was holding me back and that, if I didn't find something better, then I might have to stop."

At a Juvenile Diabetes Research Fund walk-a-thon that year, Hall-Harnden noticed a booth sponsored by the company that makes the tubeless Omnipod.

"My doctor had told me there were no other options for an insulin pump," she recalls. "I went back to him and told him, 'hey, this is what I need.' Even then, my parents and I had to fight with him about it."

BOX 3.1

Learning How to Use an Insulin Pump

- Insulin pumps serve as a sophisticated method to deliver insulin (usually regular or fast-acting insulins such as lispro or aspart).

- Traditional pumps deliver insulin from the pump to an infusion site typically on the abdomen or upper buttocks or thighs via plastic tubing.

- The Omnipod is a tubeless pump that delivers insulin from a pod that is often placed on the abdomen or upper arms.

- Pumps are programmed to give a basal insulin (a steady dose of background insulin) and bolus insulin (a burst of insulin to help cover glucose rises that happen after meals).

- Bolus insulin dosing includes two components: insulin to cover the amount of carbohydrates ingested (carbohydrate counting or "carbohydrate ratio") and also insulin to correct the premeal insulin (correctional scale or "insulin sensitivity").

- Traditional pumps may be removed for exercise events if the event is short in duration and glucose is monitored.

- All types of pumps allow for "temporary" basal rates to be programmed. This typically is a reduction of the background insulin rate for a few hours in relation to the exercise session to help reduce the risk of hypoglycemia (low glucose).

- Newer pumps that are "integrated" with sensors (use sensor data to augment/adjust insulin delivery) typically have "exercise" settings that tell the algorithm to adjust to a higher glucose target during exercise to help reduce the risk of hypoglycemia (low glucose).

— Expert Commentary —

Many exciting technologies are available that have made day-to-day management of diabetes less cumbersome. Further, technological advances have greatly facilitated many athletes with diabetes to excel in all types and levels of sports. Insulin pumps are commonly used by people with diabetes (Box 3.1).

Continuous glucose monitors (CGMs) can also be effective tools to closely follow your daily glucose patterns and negate the need to interrupt your physical activity with finger sticks. The Dexcom sensors are usually worn on the abdomen or back of the arm. Current versions are worn for 10 days, but future versions will likely be worn for longer periods (about 2 weeks). Readings can go automatically to a handheld device or a smartphone. Information can be shared to family or friends or coaches via their smartphones so they can monitor glucose levels. The FreeStyle Libre sensor is worn on the back of the arm for 14 days. It requires the user to engage or "swipe" their phone or handheld device over the sensor to get a glucose reading on demand. A potential downside of the Dexcom or FreeStyle Libre sensor is they could get dislodged during activities (such as wrestling, football, lacrosse, and basketball) or when working in tight spaces (such as any job that requires putting your arms into small, enclosed areas). If the sensor becomes dislodged, it can't be reused and would need to be replaced.

An alternative is the Eversense CGM System. This is an implantable sensor. However, it requires a short office-based procedure to place the sensor under the skin. Once the sensor is placed under the skin, a transmitter is placed on the skin that then relays glucose readings to a smartphone. The transmitter can easily be removed for athletics or work in tight spaces. Currently, the implantable sensor needs to be removed and replaced every 180 days.

There are some CGMs integrated with the insulin pump, such as those from Medtronic, Omnipod, or Tandem.

WILL CROSS describes his English childhood in the 1960s and 1970s as typical British stiff upper lip.

If something was wrong or there was something he didn't like, he says, his parents would ask him whether he planned to whine about it or take action. So, when 16-year-old Cross was angered to learn that his type 1 diabetes would prevent him from attending a government-sponsored three-month trek to Chile's Patagonia region, he says the response from his parents was predictable: "Well, what are you going to do about it?"

"To me, Patagonia was this place of romance and intrigue," Cross says. "It would be a difficult trip, a long way from nowhere. And I wanted to do it."

Each year, the Prince of Wales organized an expedition where teens from all over the United Kingdom applied for the opportunity to travel to an exotic land for community service, scientific exploration, and adventure. But Cross recalls the expedition's application stating clearly that people with epilepsy or diabetes would not be considered for the journey.

Cross had lived with diabetes for six years. By then, he had learned enough about his condition—and his own determination—that he was confident in his ability to keep up with his peers on the Chilean adventure.

To appeal his disqualification, young Will went straight to the top.

"I wrote a letter to Prince Charles," recalls Cross. "I told him we all have challenges, and this is mine."

In his letter, Cross explained that, despite diabetes, he was physically fit, he'd excelled in sports, and was up to any challenge the expedition presented.

Even before his diabetes diagnosis, Cross's early childhood and adolescence had been full of health problems.

As a toddler, Cross had a kidney ailment that his doctors treated with a powerful steroid for six months at a time. For 10 years, he'd spend half the year as an energetic kid whose kidneys didn't function properly and the other half bloated and sluggish. Cross says he wonders if his own diabetes was at all related to the kidney disease and its treatment so early in his life.

BOX 3.2

Special Considerations
for Diabetes Management While on the Go

- Traveling requires lots of planning. If you have diabetes, this adds an extra layer of complexity in packing your bag.

- Excessive exercise increases the risk of low blood glucose episodes. Make sure you have sources of fast-acting glucose to treat hypoglycemia. Juice boxes with apple or orange juice are quick sources of sugar. Oral glucose tablets are also easy to pack.

- If multiple days of activity are planned, think ahead with regard to meal planning. Concession stands or fast-food restaurants might not have available proper nutrition to refuel you between events and prevent hyperglycemia.

- Insulin becomes ineffective at very high or low temperatures. Once a vial or pen of insulin is open, it should be stored at room temperature (typically 56° to 80°F). Plan ahead. If you will be out in the heat, insulin may need to be stored in a cooler with ice. If you are in very cold temperatures, consider where you can store the insulin so it does not get too cold.

- For overnight trips, having extra supplies, such as for testing blood glucose, can be crucial. If you use an insulin pump, having backup insulin pens to use if anything happens to your pump is critical. Discuss making these kinds of transitions with your health provider so a pump failure does not derail your competition.

"I realize now that I had a lot of anger," Cross says about his health as a young child. "I think anyone with a lifelong condition goes through those feelings of denial and bargaining and, eventually, acceptance. Part of mine was, I was just pissed off."

Cross's letter persuaded Prince Charles.

"I got a letter back from [Buckingham] Palace telling me I'd made a good case and that they'd give me a shot," says Cross. "It was a highlight of my life."

The last three weeks of the Patagonian adventure went a little haywire, Cross recalls. His traveling group ran out of food and was forced to hunt and fish for the remainder of the journey. Cross persisted and finished the trip, despite needing to ration his insulin to two or three units a day.

More physically and mentally challenging than Cross expected, the Patagonia adventure set the course for much of the rest of his athletic and endurance endeavors.

Cross speaks at diabetes conferences around the world, but he avoids support groups and communities dedicated to sharing experiences.

"I respect the fact that some people get a lot out of discussion and sharing," says Cross. "I don't. I'm not really a group person. That's just my personality."

"Mountaineering is a lonely endeavor," Cross says. "I sort of enjoy the solitude. I focus on the climbing. I mean, I don't mind suffering alone. That's what mountaineering is, really."

He says he enjoys learning from researchers and physicians at the conferences.

"The data and the American Diabetes Association research, I love that stuff. I get a lot out of that. But no, I don't go to diabetes groups."

Cross and his fellow climber Sébastien Sasseville both approach their diabetes similar to the way they approach their athletic pursuits: alone.

"Diabetes has been a magnifying glass for me," says Sasseville. "It's helped me see stuff about myself that was already there."

He learned the ropes of diabetes management more or less on his own, through trial and error. He read what he could find and taught himself to eat healthier and get more exercise. Sasseville believes his approach spared his family a lot of heartache.

"When I told them I had diabetes, they were definitely sad," says Sasseville. "But then we all just said, 'OK, see you next weekend.'"

— *Expert Commentary* —

Times have changed from the 1970s when Will Cross wanted to do a government-sponsored trek to Chile's Patagonia region. But despite the fact that his story took place over 40 years ago, discrimination for people with diabetes unfortunately still occurs in the twenty-first century. Although not as exciting as Cross's three-month trek, equally important to those with diabetes is the ability to secure and maintain employment—without their diabetes getting in the way. Unfortunately, people with diabetes are not always treated fairly in the workplace. They may be overlooked for new jobs or promotions. This type of employment discrimination typically happens when a supervisor is unsure about what diabetes is or how it is treated. Educating the employer or supervisor can be helpful to prevent this from happening.

A diagnosis of diabetes can make employment more difficult in a small number of professions that require waivers or exemptions (such as the military, law enforcement, or aviation). But, in general, the Americans with Disabilities Act requires all employers to generally support the needs of people with diabetes in the workplace. In 2020, the first person with type 1 diabetes was granted a commercial pilot's license by the Federal Aviation Administration. Before this time, no insulin-treated person with diabetes was certified to pilot commercially in the United States but times are slowly changing. There are many special considerations for people with diabetes while on the go (Box 3.2).

Cross pushed the limits that had been placed before him for people with diabetes, and the future should continue to see fewer barriers across all areas of employment and opportunity of people with diabetes.

IN MAY 2008, Sébastien Sasseville climbed to the summit of Mount Everest, 29,035 feet above sea level, where springtime midday temperatures average about ⁻15°F.

Four years later, he completed a five-day footrace across the Egyptian portion of the Sahara Desert. Sasseville carried all his own food, water, and supplies across 155 miles of sand. When he crossed the finish line at the famous pyramids of Giza, he finished 21st of 134 runners.

And on a snowy February morning in 2014, Sasseville laced up his sneakers and ran from one end of Canada to the other.

The Quebec native decided to use a trans-Canadian run to raise awareness and research funds for type 1 diabetes. The nine-and-a-half-month journey from St. John's, Newfoundland, to Vancouver, British Columbia, spanned approximately 4,500 miles.

Each endeavor required every shred of strength, energy, and determination that Sasseville could summon. But when he talks about exhaustion, he doesn't mention Everest, the Sahara, or 170 marathons across Canada. He talks about trying to be perfect.

Someone who's never spoken with him could easily mistake Sasseville as a driven, single-minded obsessive to whom any kind of failure is foreign. But he insists that's not the case, adding that diabetes has taught him a certain kind of patience.

"When I was first diagnosed, I thought I had to beat diabetes," he says. "I wanted to fight it and win."

He obsessed over his blood sugar numbers and aimed for perfection. But in time, Sasseville says he came to learn that acceptance of the disease was a far better approach. Maybe he didn't need to be perfect to be happy and to live the life he wanted.

"I mean, it's not like diabetes is suddenly going to go away," he says. "It took me a few years, but I finally realized that striving to be perfect all the time is an exhausting way to live."

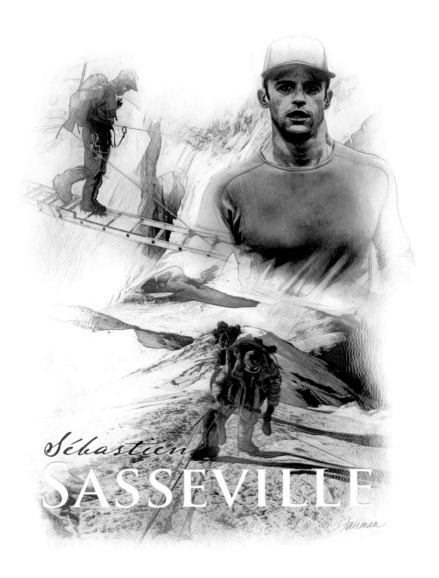

Sébastien Sasseville

SASSEVILLE

Sébastien Sasseville, Canadian mountain climber and
distance runner who summited Mount Everest and ran across Canada:
*"I've used [diabetes] as a purpose, a reason to do these difficult things. . . .
I have a disease that forces me to live a healthy life.
I want to figure out my full potential and see what I can do."*

He says his run across Canada taught him a lot about patience in managing his diabetes.

"That wasn't easy," he says, in an understatement. "I mean, between the preparation and the run itself, that was my job for about a year, right?"

Sasseville expected his diabetes to behave pretty much as it always did during his training. But he says the disease presented different challenges every day as he ran the rocky hills of Newfoundland, Quebec, and Ontario; across the prairies of Alberta, Manitoba, and Saskatchewan; and all the way to the mountains of British Columbia, finishing at Vancouver's Stanley Park, overlooking Vancouver Island and the Pacific Ocean.

Five or six days a week, Sasseville would run 12 miles in the morning and another 12 miles after lunch. He'd stop in cities along the way, doing media interviews to promote fundraising for diabetes research.

"Every day was different," he recalls. "The minute I kind of had it right, I'd get more insulin resistant. Or less insulin resistant. Or I gained a few pounds during a five-day stop in Toronto."

"You can never stop thinking about it and asking what's going to work today," he says. "That was my approach, all the way across Canada. I'd ask myself 'what's my diabetes equation today?' Because it's not a recipe; it's an equation."

Nutrition, temperature, fatigue level: essentially, Sasseville had to sort out these and all other variables that a working pancreas would take care of.

"Every day, whether you're running across the country or just living your life, there are variables. It's up to you to understand the impact of each variable in the equation."

Sasseville also has competed in numerous Ironman Triathlons and other extreme endurance competitions. From time to time, he says, he has encountered race organizers who were skeptical that a person with diabetes should undertake such a grueling physical challenge.

"It's understandable," he says. Ironman, for instance, is owned by a for-profit company. Sasseville says it's reasonable for a company that organizes races to be concerned about a racer with diabetes perhaps getting injured or ill during the competition.

"I felt it was my own responsibility to convince them that I could do it," he says. "It's my job to be well-controlled and to show up with support from health care professionals. I made it a point to patiently answer every question the organizers had."

Patience is a theme in Sasseville's life. He maintains his positive attitude about diabetes and most other life challenges well enough to earn his living as a corporate motivational speaker who specializes in the business field of change management.

"I almost feel guilty that I didn't have a depressed phase, where I struggled to cope," he says. "And I don't want to give anyone a cheesy line that success is only about attitude. It's hard. And it takes work. But we've been to space with diabetes. We've been to the Olympics and to the top of Mount Everest. Every single sport has a professional athlete with diabetes. We can do whatever we decide we want to do."

Sasseville points to scientific, medical, and technological advances in the field of diabetes.

"Thirty years ago, we didn't have fast-acting insulin. We didn't have good tools to measure our glucose. We didn't have insulin pumps," he says. "I can't even imagine what we'll have in 5, 10, or 20 years."

He's pretty sure that, had he not had diabetes, he wouldn't have become an endurance athlete.

"I've used it as a purpose, a reason to do these difficult things," he explains. "I have a disease that forces me to live a healthy life. I want to figure out my full potential and see what I can do."

— *Expert Commentary* —

Patience. This is a virtue that is so important for someone with diabetes. New situations will present themselves all the time—whether it is running across Canada, adjusting to a new work shift, altering insulin when traveling time zones, or having to bolus mealtime insulin for your mother-in-law's special meatloaf dinner. Learning about how different situations may affect your diabetes is important. Sébastien Sasseville clearly is an excellent learner. He had no way of precisely knowing how the heat of the Sahara Desert or the altitude of Mount Everest would impact his blood glucose. He researched these situations and spoke to as many people with similar experiences, but this list of people had to be very small. Ultimately, he needed to be patient and respond to the changes he saw. He was able to lean on his prior experiences to help him as well. Clearly, he was more prepared for these adventures after training and reflecting on what he learned about his diabetes during the training.

The same holds true in all walks of life. Moving from day shift to night shift might seem like no big deal other than just some sleep deprivation. But with diabetes this will likely take pre-planned adjustments in basal rates or the timing of basal injections or oral medications for people with type 2 diabetes. Things might not go perfectly smoothly the first night or the second. But constantly looking at feedback and what have you learned and how you can adjust further is the key to success. A common sentiment from people with diabetes goes like this: "I did everything the same. Ate the same foods. Did the same activities. Gave the same medicine. But still my blood sugars were vastly different . . ." This is where having the patience that Sasseville notes is so important. Being perfect all the time is not possible. But learning from each experience is possible and crucial to good control.

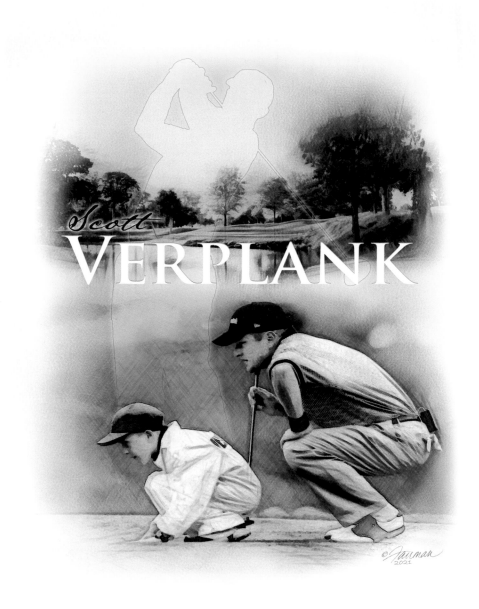

Scott Verplank, American professional golfer who has played on the
Professional Golfers Association (PGA) and PGA Champions tours:
*"I was one of the best golfers in the world in my early 20s because I had diabetes . . .
the disease forced me to be mature."*

SINCE EARNING HIS PGA Tour card in 1986, Scott Verplank has won millions and finished in the top 10 in all four of golf's major tournaments.

On a drizzly late Sunday afternoon the year before he turned pro, a 21-year-old Verplank was tied with tour veteran Jim Thorpe after four rounds at the Western Open near Chicago. The Dallas native would soon graduate from NCAA golf powerhouse Oklahoma State University, where he earned All-American honors all four years. Heading into the weekend's open tournament, Verplank was playing the best golf of his life.

But no amateur golfer had won the Western Open since 1910. And it had been nearly 30 years since anyone but a pro won any event on the PGA Tour. Heading into a sudden-death tiebreaker with the 36-year-old Thorpe, Verplank felt nervous for the first time in the tournament.

Both players saved par on the first playoff hole, but each missed the fairway off the next tee, leaving long second shots from the rough. Thorpe's ball landed on the right fringe, just off the 17th green. Verplank's shot stopped on the fairway, short of the putting surface.

The young Texan's pitch shot bounced gently on the green, settling five feet downhill from the pin. Thorpe, rain dripping from the bill of his visor, sent his chip shot skidding 15 feet past the hole. He two-putted for a bogey.

A historic championship within reach, Verplank faced precisely the kind of putt every golfer loves: slightly uphill, just a few feet from the hole. He stood over his ball and asked himself a rhetorical question.

"How many straight-in, uphill putts have you made in your life?"

With a firm tap, he rolled the ball directly into the hole for the win. But don't ask him to describe it.

"I saw it go over the lip and I went blank," Verplank told reporters after the tournament. "I don't even remember it going in."

Verplank talks about a time 12 years earlier when he "went blank" in a much more serious and dangerous way.

At age 9, his mother took him to a doctor with flu symptoms. Sure enough, the doctor told them, the kid's got the flu. But the illness worsened and stopped looking like an ordinary flu. A visit to a different doctor revealed more than just a viral infection. The physician told Verplank's mother she needed to get young Scott to Dallas Presbyterian Hospital right away.

"My parents didn't know what was wrong," says Verplank. "They just knew I wasn't getting better."

He remembers a harrowing trip to the hospital.

"In the car, I was feeling terrible. Honestly, I thought I was having a heart attack. I had chest pain and my breathing was really heavy."

He doesn't remember much after that.

"I was in a coma for a few days," he says. "I woke up and the people in the hospital showed me how to give myself an [insulin] shot using an orange. That was kind of it."

"Medicine and technology were so different then," says Verplank. "There was a whole lot of guessing. You'd test your glucose with urine, not blood."

— Expert Commentary —

Around the time that Scott Verplank was a child, most people with type 1 diabetes used animal-derived insulin from the pancreases of pigs or cows, also known as pork or beef insulin. That insulin frequently contained a lot of impurities. Human insulin was first approved in the United States in 1982, and now many synthetic insulins are available and commonly used in both type 1 and type 2 diabetes.

To monitor glucose at home, urine testing was likely the only testing available during Verplank's childhood. Home blood glucose meters and finger sticks were not in widespread use until the 1980s. The availability of CGMs for personal use did not occur until the twenty-first century.

Having the self-awareness to know what glucose highs and lows feel like, to know what and when to eat, and to know when to rest are all important pieces of good diabetes management. Learning them takes time and patience.

Even the most successful athletes need time to adjust and to find out what works and what doesn't. Little by little, good diabetes management leads to even better diabetes management.

Chapter 4

Self-Care in Diabetes

How can I prevent complications?

WHEN PEOPLE WHO HAVE type 1 diabetes are diagnosed as children, often parents and other family members have an active role in helping them to take care of their disease. But what about people diagnosed during adulthood? Who helps them learn how to interpret their glucose numbers? Or inject themselves with insulin? Or cook the right meals? Even many health-conscious people report that they learned diabetes self-care largely on their own.

"I was diagnosed on a Friday," recalls Monique Hanley, an Australian cyclist and an advocate for women's sports in her country. She got the news from her doctor while she was a 19-year-old college student. "They showed me how to give myself injections and then they sent me home."

A brand-new diagnosis of an autoimmune disease that will affect every day of the rest of your life is no small matter, even in an era when diabetes research and technology make new strides all the time.

Children can rely on their parents to help them with new diagnoses and to form the important habits they'll need to stay on top of diabetes throughout their lives. That can mean things like parents administering insulin injections and buying and preparing food that's appropriate for kids with diabetes.

But an adult diagnosis of type 1 diabetes can be a unique experience. While no one needs to feel that their life is over, the diagnosis will necessitate developing new skills in daily self-management, and it may require a certain amount of compassion and empathy from the health care professional who delivers the news.

Growing up on a dairy farm in rural Victoria, Australia, Hanley says she and her siblings learned an important lesson early in life.

"At our house, the toilets were outdoors. So, all four of us kids learned very early in life that you go before bed and then hold on until morning. Our bladders were like steel!"

So, it struck Hanley as unusual when, at 19 years old, the urge to urinate woke her multiple times a night.

She had just finished her rookie season in Australia's women's professional basketball league and was looking forward to a university semester abroad when she visited her doctor. The sophomore point guard was a few months from leaving for an exchange year at Ryerson University in Toronto, where she would study and play for the school's basketball team.

"When the doctor sat me down and told me I had diabetes, the first thing that came into my head was 'But I'm going to Canada. Are people with diabetes allowed to travel?'"

Her physician assured her that travel and athletics would be fine; but that's where her diabetes education ended.

The day after learning she would live the rest of her life with diabetes and started treatment for diabetes, Hanley played a game of netball, a modified version of basketball popular in Commonwealth nations. In Australia, it's common for teams from rural towns to play one another in informal weekend pickup netball games. After an especially productive first half, it was time for one of Hanley's first-ever finger sticks to check her blood sugar.

"I hadn't told anyone about my diagnosis," she recalls. "I mean, I didn't know what to tell them. I felt like a failure. Or like I was impure or something."

"So, at halftime, I thought I'd check my sugar in my car, away from all the other players."

She followed the directions she'd learned at her doctor's office the day before. Hanley pricked her finger, got a blood sample, and tested her sugar. Her glucose level was 6.0 mmol/L, or 106 mg/dl. It's one thing to have accurate data from blood glucose test. But it's another thing to know what to do as a result.

"I remember looking at the number and thinking I have no idea what to do with that information," she says. "The moment overwhelmed me."

Disoriented and afraid, Hanley got out of her car and told her coach she couldn't play the second half.

"The team was a bit flabbergasted because I'd been having a blinder of a game," she says, using an expression that translates, roughly, to "on a roll." She gave the coach her jersey, apologized, and returned to her car.

"I just sat there, in the car. I didn't know what to do or who to talk to."

Like many people whose type 1 diabetes develops during adulthood, Hanley's early management of the disease was hit or miss. Her exchange student–athlete adventure in Canada presented some challenges far from home.

"I learned by process of failure," she says with a laugh. "First, I lost my finger-pricker somewhere over there. I'd say that, in Canada, I learned a lot of life skills about how to survive diabetes when things go wrong."

Hanley recalls a Caribbean island trip with her teammates that turned into a hunt for the type of insulin needed before meals. Her Ryerson University team had a week-long training camp in Barbados shortly before the season opened.

"And I didn't pack enough insulin," she says. "A few days into the trip, I was like, 'I don't have any short-acting insulin left.' I ended up going to pharmacies and hospitals, looking all over for some," in a country where she had no prescription.

Her search proved futile.

"I didn't know what to do," Hanley says. "The short answer, though, is I just didn't eat much for the last few days and I just kept using my long-acting insulin until the trip back to Toronto."

Hanley's basketball talent carried her through the season in Canada. But a return to professional basketball proved trickier.

During her first season, which happened before her diabetes diagnosis, Hanley was a reserve who played only a few minutes a game to rest the starters. As she and her teammates trained for a new season, Hanley's coaches expected her to be the team's main point guard.

Preseason practices were grueling. Sprints, drills, and more sprints were exactly what you'd expect as a pro basketball player. But for the first time in Hanley's life, she struggled to keep up with her teammates. She experienced a significant drop in energy.

Feeling sluggish and exhausted in practice, Hanley found herself cutting corners—something she'd never done. Because her point guard position didn't require her to do much under the basket, she found a way to shave significant steps during practice scrimmages.

"Instead of running the full length of the basketball court, I started just running between the 3-point lines," she recalls. "I didn't have the energy, so I started 'cheating' a little."

Managing the pressure of playing professionally, while still learning how diabetes affected her body and her performance, lessened much of Hanley's enthusiasm for basketball.

Despite her role as starting point guard, Hanley's fire for the sport was diminishing along with her energy. A few weeks before the start of the season, Hanley decided she was done with basketball. She says her team's indifference toward her diabetes factored heavily in her decision to say goodbye to the sport she'd played since childhood.

"I didn't get much support from coaches or teammates. I thought, 'That's it. I'm done,'" she says. "I just decided I didn't want to do it anymore."

Freed from the rigors and inflexibility of team sports, and because inactivity wasn't part of her plans, Hanley searched for a new athletic pursuit. It turned out she didn't need to look far.

Hanley had always loved riding a bicycle. But she'd never considered riding competitively, even though her hometown is a hotbed of competitive cycling.

The town of Warragul sits 60 miles southeast of Melbourne, among hills and winding roads that bend around farms and livestock fields. It is home to an outdoor velodrome—an oval cycling track with two steep, 180-degree banked turns and two straightaways. The town also hosts an annual road race that draws many of the top cyclists in Australia.

"I'd always ridden a bike as a child," she says. "But it was more a way to get around than a form of exercise."

Little by little, cycling helped Hanley fall in love with sports again. She started riding long distances with a men's cycling club in Victoria.

Just as she had in basketball, Hanley experienced barriers the more serious she got about cycling. Only this time, the barriers had more to do with being a woman than with having diabetes.

"I learned early on that was a place you had to be fit enough and tough enough to hang in," she says of the training rides with a men's club. "I realized that this wasn't a space that really encouraged newcomers to the sport. If you couldn't keep up, you had a long ride home by yourself."

Soon, Hanley became not only a competitive cyclist but also an advocate, both for women's cycling in general and for athletes who have type 1 diabetes.

She founded and led an organization dedicate to making the

BOX 4.1

Diabetes Self-Management
Education and Support

All people with diabetes should participate in diabetes self-management education and support (DSMES) training upon diagnosis, and likely at other times too (such as if targets are not being met or if complications occur). DSMES is important to facilitate the knowledge and skills needed for good diabetes self-care. Talk to your health care provider or diabetes educator to learn more about available programs. These core topics are usually covered:

- Pathophysiology and treatments available for diabetes
- Healthy eating
- Being active
- Medication usage
- Monitoring of glucose levels
- Preventing, detecting, and treating acute complications
  - Hypoglycemia, hyperglycemia
  - Diabetic ketoacidosis, sick days
  - Severe weather or crisis supply management/disaster preparedness
- Preventing, detecting, and treating chronic complications
  - Immunizations
  - Eye, foot, kidneys, heart
  - Dental
- Healthy coping
- Problem-solving

---

sport of cycling more welcoming to women. And she founded and led another organization to encourage people with diabetes to stay active and pursue their own athletic dreams.

Hanley's cycling achievements are astounding. She rode across Canada. She was the only woman on a team of racers that won a race across the United States, setting a new course record. And in 2003, she "chased" the Tour de France, following the famous race on her own bike, carrying with her only a tent, a sleeping bag, and her diabetes supplies.

— *Expert Commentary* —

With a new diagnosis of diabetes, it is not uncommon to feel overwhelmed. Not only are there lifestyle changes but adapting to daily finger sticks and taking medications regularly (particularly frequent insulin injections) can be daunting. For many individuals, it comes down to figuring out what works best through trial and error, such as determining which glucose level is optimal for them before starting exercise to prevent unexpected drops. At times, it may seem that even with the same daily routine the glucose levels fluctuate unexpectedly, and it is not uncommon to feel a lack of control. Good self-care in diabetes includes recognizing that some days will be better than others. The more educated an individual is about their disease, such as understanding what the numbers mean and setting realistic goals, the more empowered and motivated they may be to manage their disease at home. There are many diabetes self-management resources available (Box 4.1). Difficulties are sure to arise but being able to effectively problem-solve and maintain a positive attitude are imperative.

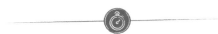

FANS WHO VISIT State Farm Arena in downtown Atlanta, Georgia, never need to wonder who was the greatest player in the history of the NBA's Atlanta Hawks.

Right outside the arena's ticket office towers a 9-ton statue of

Hawks legend Dominique Wilkins. The bronze figure captures Wilkins in mid-air, basketball in hand, poised for one of his soaring, one-handed windmill dunks that rattled NBA backboards in the 1980s and 1990s.

After a three-year All-Southeast Conference and All-American career at the University of Georgia, Wilkins played 16 seasons in the NBA and two more in European professional leagues. A nine-time NBA All-Star, he averaged nearly 25 points per game in his NBA career—14th on the all-time list.

The 6-foot, 8-inch Wilkins led the league in scoring in the 1985–1986 season (30.3 points per game), guiding the Hawks to the Eastern Conference Semifinals, where they lost to eventual champion Boston Celtics.

"The Human Highlight Film" won the NBA Slam Dunk Contest in 1985 and 1990. He was inducted into the Basketball Hall of Fame in 2006, seven years after his playing career ended.

Wilkins has served since 2004 as the Hawks' vice president of basketball. In 2007, the team made him the lead analyst on its 82 regular-season television broadcasts.

In addition to his legendary talent, Wilkins was known during his playing days for his durability and conditioning. Before suffering a ruptured Achilles tendon halfway through his 10th NBA season, Wilkins missed only 18 of the Hawks' 738 games from 1982 to 1992. The injury likely cost him a spot on the legendary 1992 US Olympic "Dream Team," alongside Michael Jordan, Magic Johnson, Larry Bird, Charles Barkley, and other stars of the day.

And, at 32 years old, less than a year after the Achilles injury, Wilkins picked up where he left off, averaging 30 points per game in the Hawks' 1992–1993 season. He also played on the US National Team in 1994's World Championships in Canada, averaging 12.6 points per game as the "Dream Team II" finished the international tournament 8 and 0, winning by an average margin of 37 points.

In June 1999, after half a season with the Orlando Magic, Wilkins was finally ready to retire from the grind of the NBA.

But not long after his retirement, the telltale signs of frequent urination and general fatigue started to surface. His vision got blurry, and he began wearing eyeglasses. Though his father and grandfather both died from complications of diabetes, Wilkins felt his years of obsessive conditioning meant he wouldn't develop the disease.

During his first year away from basketball, Wilkins was out for dinner one evening with his younger brother Gerald, who himself played 13 years in the NBA. Gerald noticed that his brother wasn't quite himself.

"I didn't feel sick," says Wilkins. "I just felt 'off.'"

He visited his physician, and after routine blood work, Wilkins says his doctor gave him the old "good news–bad news" routine.

"He said the good news is you're not dying yet," Wilkins recalls. "I was, like, 'What does *that* mean?' He said, don't get alarmed but you have type 2 diabetes. We need to make a lifestyle change right now."

Unlike type 1 diabetes, type 2 diabetes doesn't destroy the cells that make insulin. Instead, people who have type 2 diabetes don't adequately respond to insulin the way their bodies need to.

Wilkins' recollection of "feeling off" is common among people before a diagnosis of type 2 diabetes. The gradual nature of the body's growing resistance to the hormone that regulates blood glucose can produce run-down, quick-to-fatigue symptoms that accompany hyperglycemia (high blood glucose).

Type 2 diabetes is far more common than type 1. In 2020, the CDC estimated that, while about 1.9 million Americans have type 1 diabetes, more than 35.4 million Americans were living with type 2 diabetes, either diagnosed or undiagnosed. Risk factors for type 2 diabetes include family history, carrying excess weight, inactivity, age, and race or ethnicity.

The risk isn't just about excess weight. It's also about where one carries excess weight. Abdominal fat puts people at greater risk of diabetes.

Wilkins was never anyone's idea of overweight. Even a year after his playing career ended, he didn't carry a lot of fat in his midsection. But his family history and genetic predisposition meant that eventually his body might need some help regulating its blood sugar.

Risk factors for diabetes affect everyone differently; some people go on to develop the disease while others do not, and this often depends on the presence of other lifestyle factors such as physical inactivity and diet, as well.

During his playing years, between practices, training, and the long NBA season schedule and postseason, Wilkins ate whatever he wanted and never gained weight.

"Once life slowed down and I wasn't training like that anymore, I found out I had a problem that a lot of Americans have. It's harder to burn off those calories. And my body couldn't handle sugar like it had for years."

Wilkins learned that a special favorite of his would now be off limits.

"I had to cut back or quit eating some foods that I'd always eaten," he says. "But for me, orange juice was a tough one."

Wilkins had consumed orange juice in huge quantities his whole life. It's natural, and it's full of vitamin C and potassium. Perfect, right?

Nope. Despite its vitamins and minerals, orange juice contains about as much sugar as Coca-Cola. And it has more calories.

"When somebody's blood sugar gets low, what's the first thing they're given? Orange juice," says Wilkins. "It'll raise your sugar to the roof."

Wilkins' doctor suggested he drop the juice and switch to water. He did, and he hasn't looked back.

"I haven't had orange juice in 21 years," he laughs. "Now I drink a lot of water during a day. Over a gallon. I tell people that's one of the keys to managing diabetes: drinking a lot of water. Make sure you take your medication the right way and drink a lot of water."

Wilkins says he took diabetes seriously immediately. He cut back on sugar and made sure to stay active.

"I lost 35 pounds in the three months after I found out I had diabetes," he says. "And I've kept that weight off for all these years."

He describes the transition to living with diabetes in the matter-of-fact manner he used to talk about his basketball accomplishments.

"Once I accepted that I have diabetes and that it's going to mean I have to pay attention to my health for the rest of my life, it wasn't that hard of an adjustment. I just think of it as another opponent I compete with."

Despite his job as an executive and broadcaster with the Hawks, Wilkins says he doesn't play much ball anymore.

"I still shoot around with my son from time to time," he says. "But I'm just always busy. Always doing something. A lot of people think you have to join a gym or something, but your workout is right outside your front door. You just got to keep yourself physically moving."

Wilkins travels with the team to its 41 road games each season. The travel, he says, doesn't mean it's time to ignore diabetes. Away from home, he could easily fall into unhealthy eating habits. But the team's players, coaches, and staff all need to eat healthy too.

"Our team has breakfast, lunch, and dinner all set up for us in our hotels," he explains. "They serve really good and really healthy meals. So, there's a lot to choose from."

Since the NBA season stretches through the winter months, much of the Hawks' travel is to cold-weather cities like Toronto, Milwaukee, and Chicago. For those trips, Wilkins gets his exercise in gyms at the home team's arena.

But western cities are different, he says.

"Out there, we walk a lot," he says. "There are quite a few of us from the team who'll get up early and take a long walk" in Los Angeles, Phoenix, San Antonio, and other NBA cities that don't freeze in January and February.

Along with strict adherence to the medication his doctor prescribed, the weight loss and lifestyle adjustment that Wilkins made during his first year away from basketball has allowed him to stay healthy and enjoy a long career doing what he loves.

He says he noticed a critical difference only a few weeks after he started taking medication and changed his diet.

"I rolled over in bed one morning and I could see the alarm clock, clear as a bell," Wilkins says. As he managed diabetes, his vision improved markedly.

Wilkins says that, when he talks to people about managing diabetes, he urges them to stick with it.

"I see a lot of people who, when they start doing well, the first thing they do is cut back," he says. "That's the wrong thing to do. You've got to stay on course."

— Expert Commentary —

Type 2 diabetes accounts for the majority of diabetes worldwide (about 90%–95%) and type 1 diabetes accounts for about 5%. For people with type 2 diabetes, focusing on lifestyle changes is critical to good self-care. Persons who are overweight or obese are much more likely to develop type 2 diabetes because excess fat makes the body more resistant to the effects of insulin; an accumulation of abdominal fat (often leading to an increased waist circumference) is particularly concerning. As a result, insulin cannot lower blood glucose levels as effectively. Over time, prediabetes may occur; this is a high-risk state where blood glucose levels are higher than normal but not yet high enough to be classified as diabetes. However, without intensive lifestyle

TABLE 4.1.

Recommended routine preventive care measures

DAILY OR WEEKLY	CHECK EVERY 3–6 MONTHS	CHECK ONCE A YEAR
Take prescribed medications and check blood glucose levels at home at prescribed frequency (*usually 1–4 times/day*)	Visit with your health care provider	Dilated eye exam by eye care professional
Check blood pressure at home (*if recommended for hypertension*)	A1C level	Cholesterol test*
Visually inspect feet for sores, cuts, redness, or changes to the skin or nails (*especially if you have nerve damage*)	Visit dentist twice a year	Comprehensive foot exam with podiatrist*
Exercise regularly (*150 minutes per week of aerobic exercise; 1–2 muscle strengthening sessions/ week*)	See dietitian and/or nurse educator as needed	Urine microalbumin protein test and blood test for kidney function, electrolytes, liver function, etc.*
Healthy diet (*weight loss goal of approximately 5%*)		Routine yearly vaccinations (for influenza, for example). Pneumonia and hepatitis B series are also often recommended as one-time doses.

*As recommended by the health care provider. May need to be checked more often in some individuals, especially after starting a new medication or after recent dose changes.

modifications to diet and exercise and weight loss (usually the goal is ~5%), diabetes can eventually develop. Consequently, meeting with a dietitian and nurse educator is important as part of a comprehensive care plan for diabetes. Recommendations for exercise in diabetes including 30 minutes of moderate-intensity aerobic exercise (such as brisk walking, jogging, or biking) five days a week and a few bouts of muscle-strengthening exercises (such as lifting weights) a few days per week. It is important to ensure that routine preventive measures are followed to prevent the development of complications with any type of diabetes (Table 4.1).

WHEN DOCTORS TOLD Cathy Reese her 7-year-old son Riley has type 1 diabetes, she followed a trial-and-error path familiar to anyone who's learned that they or a family member has the disease. Finding the right physician, finding low-carbohydrate snacks that a 7-year-old might actually eat, deciding what equipment and technology to use—just one of these decisions might feel overwhelming. But solving problems one at a time was a luxury the Reese family didn't have.

Reese, head coach of women's lacrosse at the University of Maryland, remembers the days and months after Riley got his diagnosis.

"I remember wondering, 'how are we ever going to figure this out?'"

It's one thing to motivate and care for yourself after a diabetes diagnosis. But when your child is the one with diabetes, it's another story altogether.

A little bit at a time, says Reese, after late nights and lots of tears, she and her husband came to terms with young Riley's diabetes.

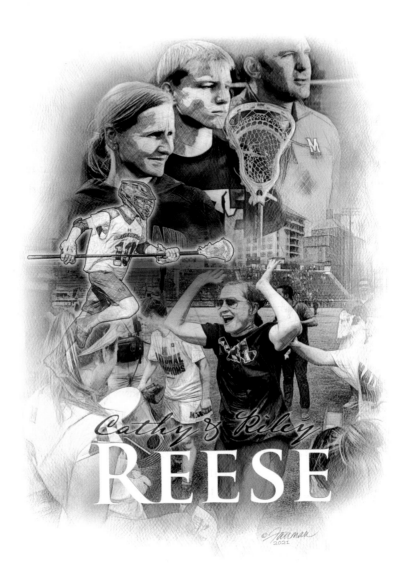

Cathy and Riley Reese, head coach and 5-time national champion
with the University of Maryland women's lacrosse team,
and her son who plays on the men's lacrosse team at the same college:
*"I remember wondering, 'how are we ever going to figure this out?'
It's just one of those things . . . we can handle this."*

"It's just one of those things," she remembers thinking. "We can handle this."

When Reese discusses her son's diabetes, she uses an unexpected pronoun: we.

We were diagnosed. *We* started using an insulin pump. *We* were hospitalized on Super Bowl Sunday. While Reese isn't conscious of her pronoun use, it's indicative of the deep empathy and active involvement in their child's health care that parents of kids with diabetes often have.

Six months or so after Riley's diagnosis, Reese began searching for a new endocrinologist. Not because the first one wasn't good, she says, but because "you need to find an endocrinologist you like and connect with. This is a long-haul disease."

Living in the Baltimore–Washington corridor offers the Reese family many options when it comes to Riley's care. The area is home to several of the nation's top research universities and hospitals, as well as the National Institutes of Health.

But driving to weekday doctor appointments on some of America's most congested highways factored into the family's decision of where Riley might be best served. Cathy and her husband both work full-time jobs and are committed to encouraging all four of their children to not only play sports but also have full kid experiences.

Still, Reese says she and her husband traded the convenience of having a pediatric diabetes specialist near their home for the confidence of taking Riley to an academic children's medical center with a large type 1 diabetes program. While not especially far from their home, the hospital is not an easy drive.

Despite the hustle and the traffic, Reese has no regrets about the family's decision.

"Our doctor has been fantastic," says Reese. "She's fun, for one thing. If you're going to be seeing an endocrinologist, I think you really need to be comfortable" with the selection.

"For another thing, it's just a different world" at an academic hospital.

In fact, soon after their switch to the children's hospital, Riley's endocrinologist determined that he also has celiac disease, which is more common in people with diabetes.

"That makes his having diabetes even more complicated," says Reese.

Like type 1 diabetes, celiac is a disease of the immune system. People who have it need to avoid eating foods that contain gluten, a protein found in wheat and other grains. Most people who have celiac experience serious gastrointestinal distress when they eat foods like bread, pasta, or even certain condiments, such as soy sauce or ketchup.

But, more often than not, celiac shows no symptoms in type 1 patients. They don't have the stomach pain or severe diarrhea or constipation that typically strikes celiac sufferers when they eat foods with gluten in them.

Reese says Riley "could eat a bagel and you wouldn't know anything was wrong."

A lack of symptoms, however, does not mean a person with celiac should eat whatever they want. For people with asymptomatic celiac disease, it's important to stick to a gluten-free diet. Even without the unpleasant symptoms, gluten still damages certain cells in the small intestine and can be associated with other autoimmune diseases, like rheumatoid arthritis.

Soon after his celiac diagnosis, Riley accompanied the Maryland women's lacrosse team on a trip to play a late-afternoon Saturday game at the University of North Carolina. On their way back to College Park after the game, a 14–11 loss for Reese's Terps, the team stopped for dinner at a Chapel Hill restaurant. While the players and other coaches and staff ordered their meals, Reese scanned the menu for something her son could eat that wouldn't send his blood sugar soaring and would comply with his need to avoid gluten.

"There literally wasn't anything else he could eat, so I ordered him the filet mignon," Reese laughs. "In a group of athletes who'd just played an NCAA lacrosse game, the eight-year-boy's dinner cost more than anyone else's!"

As much as parents and other loved ones care about their children, management of diabetes is ultimately up to the person who has the disease. Cathy Reese and her husband keep close watch on Riley's diabetes, but they also allow him room to learn about it himself.

Riley recognizes when his blood sugar is out of balance and knows what to do. No matter what sport he's playing, he checks his sugar before his pregame warmups begin.

"The basal [rate] keeps me on a pretty steady range," Riley says. "I won't usually check my sugar during a game unless I'm feeling really bad."

He wears his pod that delivers insulin on his hip during games, but he finds a continuous glucose monitor uncomfortable and distracting. Though his mother loved it, Riley eventually decided the continuous monitor wasn't for him.

"It was great," says Cathy Reese. "But I became pretty psycho about it."

No matter where Riley was, his sensor would send his glucose reading to an app on his mother's mobile phone. Reese says the information "was almost too much. In the middle of a school day, I'd get an alarm or something on my phone" that Riley's sugar was low or high. Reese made frequent calls to Riley's school nurse, who pulled the boy out of classes to make sure he was OK.

"He'd say 'I'm fine, Mom!' and we'd find out it was nothing," she recalls. "At some point, we just decided it wasn't good for us. It was over the top. It's almost too much information."

While pumps and monitors have revolutionized the way many people manage their diabetes, they're not for everyone. The Reeses decided Riley was better off without a continuous glucose monitor.

For his part, Riley, now in college, says that having diabetes hasn't hindered him. He is committed to play Division I lacrosse at the same college where his mom coaches the women's lacrosse team.

"It was hard," he says, of the early years after his diagnosis. But with a teenager's shrug, he adds, "I've gotten used to it."

— *Expert Commentary* —

Parents, family members, friends, teachers, and other loved ones have a tremendous role in supporting the self-care of an individual with diabetes, especially when they are diagnosed during childhood. As a caregiver, parents also have an important role in supporting their child toward independence in managing the disease as they grow older. Finding a health care team that is aligned with the needs of the patient and the family is imperative. Learning how to navigate new situations such as eating out at restaurants or spending time with others in social interactions encompass the types of lifestyle changes that often accompany a new diagnosis of diabetes.

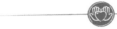

AT ITS HIGHEST LEVELS of competition, golf requires an almost surgical focus and precision. Golfers talk about the "touch" that the sport requires, a combination of strength and finesse. A well-struck shot "feels" good. The sensation in the hands and wrists when a club strikes a ball tells experienced golfers everything they need to know about the shot.

Touch and feel are so important in golf that serious players remove their golf glove before they putt, so as not to dampen the vibration and resistance they feel when putter strikes ball, however miniscule.

The last thing a golfer needs is shaky hands from a low blood glucose episode.

Scott Verplank's career as a professional golfer has depended on keeping his blood sugar well-managed. But Verplank takes that a step farther. He credits diabetes with actually improving his game.

"The disease forced me to be mature," he says. "I was one of the best golfers in the world in my early 20s *because* I had diabetes."

He says he realized at a young age that he wanted to be a pro golfer. And he knew that meant he'd need to stay healthy. So, Verplank's diabetes management verged on the obsessive.

"If my sugar's wrong, I can't play," he says in his Dallas drawl. "If I'm low, I get shaky. And if the sugar is high, I get sluggish."

Over the course of his life and career, Verplank has gotten more comfortable discussing his diabetes. But that hasn't always been the case.

"In high school and college, I was very guarded about it. I didn't want to talk about diabetes. But I checked my sugar probably 15 times a day."

Keeping his glucose levels under control has allowed Verplank to enjoy a long and lucrative career, first on the PGA Tour and later on the PGA Tour Champions, a pro circuit for players over the age of 50.

More than almost any other sport, golf is dominated by tradition and etiquette: Never walk in an opponent's field of play. Stand silent and still while others in your group are hitting. Rake the sand trap after hitting from it.

And, until the last 20 years or so, hardly anyone ate or drank while playing a round. Sure, golfers could stop in the clubhouse at the ninth hole for a snack and bathroom break. But on the course itself, it was rare to see a golfer pull anything to eat from his golf bag.

Not true for Verplank.

"In the 1980s and '90s, nobody ever ate on the golf course," he says. "Except me. Now everyone does it."

Verplank's golf bag is like a snack bar.

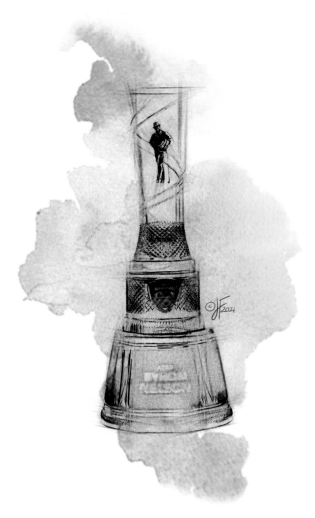

AT&T Byron Nelson PGA golf tournament trophy

"Peanut butter and jelly sandwiches, raisins, granola, Gatorade," he says. "I have it all in there."

And for good reason. While most courses insist that recreational players rent golf carts for their rounds, pro golfers walk all 18 holes. A regulation course is about 7,200 yards long—a little more than four miles. Walking that distance for a four-hour round of competitive golf without nutrition would surely cause blood sugar problems for players with diabetes.

Today, Verplank wears an insulin pump on the course. He still checks his glucose but not as often as he did in his college days. His continuous glucose monitor handles those duties now. But he says there's no handbook or set of rules for keeping his sugar steady during a tense golf tournament.

The adrenaline that every golfer's body produces at the most high-stakes moments could easily ruin Verplank's chances at finishing on the leaderboard.

A hormone secreted by the adrenal glands, adrenaline (also known as epinephrine) is an important component to the body's "fight or flight" response. It tells us to heighten our senses, keep lookout, beware of predators. Or, in Verplank's case, it instructs him to be careful of greenside bunkers and water hazards.

It also has immediate effects on blood flow, heartbeat, pupil dilation, and blood sugar levels. The pressure or stress Verplank experiences at critical moments during tournament golf leads to a release of adrenaline into his system, sending his glucose numbers soaring.

"Golf and tournament golf are two completely different sports," he says. "My sugar goes high by the second hole when I'm playing tournament golf. When I tee off on the first hole, my sugar's about 150. By the second hole, it's around 220."

It's easy to think of golf as a game where players enjoy a long stroll in the sun, stopping now and then to hit a shot. But professional golfers put enormous strain on their backs, shoulders, and wrists.

Verplank's career has been full of injuries, particularly to his joints. He's had surgeries on both elbows, as well as on his left wrist and his right thumb. But he continues to play on the Champions Tour.

"I've certainly had a lot of joint issues," he says. "I can't say for sure if they're related [to diabetes]. It's probably a combination of heavy use and diabetes. I do know that I don't heal as quickly as some people do."

Verplank says he has his own ways of keeping his diabetes under control. What to eat, how to exercise, and what kind of medicine and technology he uses are the result of a lifetime of learning about his disease and how it affects his system.

The schedule and life of a pro golfer is unique, he says. What works for one person who has diabetes probably won't work for him. He recalls traveling to Boston years ago for a six-day course on diabetes management.

"I left after the second day," he says with a mild Texas twang. "I wasn't able or going to do the regimen they recommended for me." The course instructors emphasized consistency and routine, things that were foreign to Verplank.

"I'm not an 8 to 5 guy," he says. "I might get out of bed at 5 a.m. for a 7 a.m. tee time. And the next day, I might not tee off until noon."

— *Expert Commentary* —

Scott Verplank noted that "golf" and "tournament golf" are two completely different sports in the way they might affect his diabetes. The same might be said for practicing your piano at home compared to playing Carnegie Hall or practicing parallel parking at the local high school compared to taking your driver's exam. When placed in a highly stressful situation like the final round of a major golf tournament, a normal reaction from your body is the production of stress hormones. Key among them is adrenaline, which is also called epinephrine. In addition, cortisol and growth hormone are also produced. All these hormones work in concert to raise blood glucose. In a Tuesday practice round, Verplank may see a slight rise in his glucose after teeing off. On a Sunday at the Masters when in contention, Verplank might see a dramatic rise in his glucose after the first tee. Understanding this expected response to extreme stress may better allow someone with diabetes a chance to control their glucose in this type of situation.

Understanding how changes in dietary and physical activity patterns, and also intense or stressful situations, may uniquely impact an individual's blood glucose patterns during the day is key to preventing both high and low blood glucose levels. The degree of care needed to successfully manage diabetes in childhood requires a high level of maturity and responsibility from an early age. Some persons newly diagnosed with a chronic disease may be private about their diagnosis initially while others may be more open with family and friends. In the long-term, by sharing the unique needs required to successfully self-manage diabetes with others, traditions or rules at the workplace can appropriately adapt to the changing circumstances of employees.

NO SOONER DID Doug Burns find purpose in his life than a physician advised him to abandon that purpose.

Diagnosed with type 1 diabetes at age 7, Burns was severely underweight for his age and endured one lengthy hospital stay after another.

Burns says now that he spent his childhood in a near-constant state of ketoacidosis.

When Burns's father changed jobs, the family moved from the Washington suburbs to a sleepy small town near an air force base on Mississippi's Gulf Coast.

Kicking around his new town, young Burns stumbled across a muscle magazine and discovered an instant hero: Johnny Weissmuller, an Olympic swimmer who'd later become a bodybuilder and an actor best-known for playing Tarzan in low-budget action films of the 1930s and 1940s. Glossy black-and-white photos of the

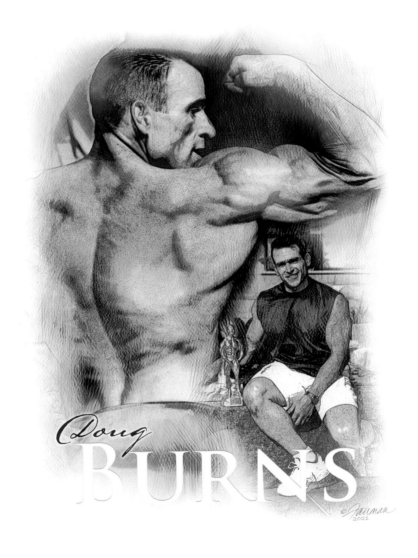

Doug

BURNS

Doug Burns, American strength athlete,
bodybuilder, and a former Natural Mr. Universe:
"I just wasn't going to stop."

low-calorie Gatorade. Always making things a little better. I just can't even imagine all they've done for me."

Perez says her mother has been involved in her diabetes management routines from day one.

"Even today, I share my Dexcom notifications with my mom's cell phone," says Perez. She'll still call me in the middle of the night, 'hey, are you eating anything?' And I'm, like, yeah, Mom, I'm fine."

Diabetes can be an isolating disease. For people like Perez, a reliable network of family, friends, medical professionals, and others serves as a lifeline for answers, help or as just a sounding board. After the initial jolts of fear and uncertainty around a diabetes diagnosis, attentive parenting can make all the difference in the ability to lead a long and healthy life.

Perez's mother, Sonja, had worked as a medical assistant in a pediatric practice for 10 years when she learned Kylee had type 1 diabetes.

"It was scary," says Sonja Perez of her daughter's diagnosis. "I'd seen a lot of kids get diagnosed with diabetes, so I was very familiar with it."

But she says that, since patients with diabetes were almost always sent to endocrinologists right away, she never had the chance to talk much with parents about dealing with the day-to-day challenges that face kids who have diabetes.

Kylee's father, Jeff, says he'd never encountered diabetes before Kylee's diagnosis.

"We definitely had more than one cram session on the Internet, just trying to learn as much as we could," he says. "I remember thinking, 'holy cow. I had no idea.'"

Sonja's familiarity with the disease didn't make it any easier to get the news. She noticed 9-year-old Kylee losing weight and feeling thirsty all the time. She mentioned the symptoms to a physician she worked with, who urged Sonja to bring Kylee in for tests.

Just as she'd feared, her daughter's diagnosis was type 1 diabetes.

"I just knew it," Sonja recalls. "I knew right away" that the disease was now a part of the Perez family.

Kylee's parents and younger sister, Briana, soon learned more about diabetes than any of them expected.

"It becomes a family disease," says Sonja. "Everybody is involved."

"Yeah, it's definitely not a one-size-fits-all situation," Jeff adds.

The Perez's emphasize that parents of kids who have diabetes need to be flexible; the disease tends to change over time.

"Any time we thought we had it figured out, a couple of months would go by and everything we thought we knew went out the window," says Jeff.

It was clear from an early age that Kylee Perez would be an athlete. Jeff and Sonja encouraged her to play any sport she wanted. In addition to softball, the northern California native spent her childhood playing soccer and basketball. Briana, who would later join her on the Bruins softball team during Kylee's senior season, also grew up playing youth sports. Thus, the Perez family spent a lot of time traveling to tournaments and watching their daughters' games.

Jeff recalls a summer softball tournament when Kylee was 11 or 12.

"The heat was just brutal. Like, 100 degrees and blazing sun," he says. "The kids were all in the dugout and the stands were packed full of families."

"We had our little mid-game testing routine that just seemed normal to us," says Jeff. "At some point, between innings, Kylee would come out of the dugout and come up to the fence and I had a small ice chest with her insulin and the rest of her supplies. Kylee just kind of stuck her arm up against the chain-link fence."

Through the metal fence, Jeff pricked his daughter's finger to get a small blood sample.

TABLE 5.1.

TABLE 5.1.
Hypoglycemia

Early signs and symptoms of hypoglycemia	Anxiety, irritability, hunger, sweating, shaking, or heart palpitations
Late signs and symptoms of hypoglycemia	Headaches, blurry vision, dizziness, confusion, seizure, or coma.
Hypoglycemia unawareness	After repeated and frequent bouts of low glucose, sometimes individuals can stop having symptoms when blood glucose levels are low. This dangerous condition can lead to no warning signs before severe consequences of hypoglycemia occur.
15/15 rule for treating hypoglycemia	If your glucose is <70 md/dl or you are experiencing symptoms of low blood glucose, consume 15 grams of fast-acting carbohydrates. Some examples are: • 6 ounces of orange or apple juice • Few hard candies • Few oral glucose tablets Chocolate candies are not a good choice as the chocolate slows digestion and absorption. Wait 15 minutes after consuming the carbohydrates. Repeat the fingerstick blood glucose check. If the glucose value is not back to normal (80–130 mg/dl), ingest another 15 grams of carbohydrates and repeat the glucose 15 minutes later. Continue to repeat this until the hypoglycemia episode has resolved.

"Everybody's eyes got really big when that needle came out," he laughs. "We definitely got a lot of looks."

Because Kylee played more than just softball, the Perez family devised similar routines for other sports. Jeff recalls, during Kylee's basketball-playing days, he or Sonja would subtly make their way behind the team bench during games. During time-outs or periods when Kylee wasn't in the game, Jeff or Sonja would have their daughter's blood test kit ready to go.

"Kylee would kind of lean back and put her arm out. One of us would test her really quick and tell her" what her glucose number was. "And then she'd throw down some apple juice or something and be fine the rest of the game."

Sonja and Jeff say their daughter's determination and strength played a key role in her taking charge of her own health. But, as a small child, those qualities presented a few parenting challenges when it came to diabetes. The parents walked a fine line between encouraging Kylee's independence and keeping a close eye on her diabetes management.

"Kylee's always wanted to do things for herself," says Sonja. "She doesn't want to bother us or her coaches or teammates, so she rarely asks for help. When she was still really young, I'd tell her to let us know what she needed. She'd say, 'Mom, I've got this!' And I'd say, 'No, Kylee, you don't got it! Not yet!'"

By the time Kylee reached high school, says Sonja, she had phone numbers and email addresses for her diabetes doctors and nurses.

"If something got out of whack and she had a question about something, there was always someone Kylee could get ahold of," Sonja says. "She wanted to take care of it herself."

Of course, parents can't be everywhere. Perez had a core of close friends and softball teammates during her teen years who helped her keep an eye on her diabetes.

"I started spending more and more time with this one group of girls," she recalls. "It was just a really close-knit group."

During high school and travel softball season, teams frequently play on consecutive days—sometimes two or even three games in one afternoon. Between practices, games, and travel, teammates spend enormous amounts of time together. Perez's teammates in her hometown in Contra County, California, came to know her very well.

"They ended up being able to tell when my sugar was higher or lower than it should be. They'd be, like, 'hey, maybe you should go test' and things. Just, like, little reminders, even if I told them I was OK. They were supportive, no matter what."

As she grew up, it became clear that Perez was going to be a force on the softball diamond. She was named the most valuable player in her high school league—after her ninth-grade season. The freshman drove in 29 runs, hit 9 home runs, stole 35 bases, and batted a gaudy .628 for the season. Even with three years of high school remaining, Perez decided she wanted to play for the winningest softball school in America: UCLA.

Perez's diligence in managing her diabetes meant she was comfortable taking charge of her own health. But she would need coaches, trainers, athletic directors, and other university officials to be aware of her chronic disease and to support decisions Perez might make based on her health, rather than strictly softball success.

Perez's father remembers the family's recruiting visit to UCLA. The softball program had kept an eye on Kylee and recruited her heavily since her freshman year of high school. The Bruins coaching staff knew just about everything there was to know about the young prospect's game on the field.

When the Perez's visited the school's legendary Westwood campus, it felt like a formality, says Jeff. Kylee wanted to play for the Bruins and the Bruins wanted Kylee. But something important was missing.

"I remember we were walking around that beautiful campus with the coaches and everything they were saying sounded great," Jeff says. "But I took just a second and pulled them aside and said sort of quietly, 'you guys know Kylee has type 1 diabetes, right?' I mean, because nobody had mentioned it so far."

Jeff describes a long pause and a glance exchanged by the coaches that suggested they did not, in fact, know that their top recruit had type 1 diabetes.

"It felt like forever," he says. "But it was probably just a second or two. Finally, [UCLA head coach Kelly Inouye-Perez] told us, 'OK. That's something we'll figure out. We'll manage it.'"

Despite being the one of the best softball players in America, Kylee Perez was still Jeff and Sonja's young adult daughter. The coach's response "was a pretty comforting thing to hear, as a parent," says Jeff. "It made us feel very comfortable" with Kylee's decision to attend and play for UCLA.

Throughout her years at the school, Kylee says her coaches and teammates made no issue of her diabetes. She appreciated her coaches' honesty and directness.

"When I got there, they told me straight up they had no idea what type 1 diabetes was," she says. "But they said they'd do their research and support me with whatever I needed."

The university's softball program lived up to its promise. Over the course of Perez's four years with the Bruins, she says her coaches and trainers were attentive and accommodating when she needed them to be.

"You know, as time progressed while I was at UCLA, [the softball staff] gained so much knowledge about diabetes that they could recognize some of my highs and lows just like my teammates. That was pretty cool."

By the end of her senior season at UCLA, Perez ranked among the storied program's all-time leaders in numerous offensive categories. She ranks third among Bruins in career hits (301), fourth in runs scored (191), and seventh in career batting average (.387). UCLA won 197 games during Perez's career and culminated each season with an appearance in the Women's College World Series.

— Expert Commentary —

Living with diabetes can be overwhelming at times. There are many lifestyle changes that are often needed, including frequent finger-stick monitoring of blood glucose levels, particularly for patients on multiple injections of insulin a day. The support of family, friends, and teammates is crucial, especially when they are also able to recognize concerning symptoms of hypoglycemia and prompt the person with diabetes to check their blood glucose levels. Many persons with diabetes treated with insulin will experience hypoglycemia (low blood glucose) at some point. Symptoms of hypoglycemia typically occur at levels of <70 md/dl (Table 5.1). Hypoglycemia can occur from taking too much insulin or eating less than expected, or a delayed meal can lead to hypoglycemia. Exercise certainly increases hypoglycemia risk by increasing insulin sensitivity in some individuals. Drinking alcohol or having an illness both increase the risk of hypoglycemia as well.

IT SEEMS UNLIKELY THAT, in the long history of the Pittsburgh Pirates, Jason Johnson was the first player in the organization with diabetes. In fact, records show that diabetes cut short the career of young Pirates shortstop Coburn Jones in 1929. But Johnson was surely among the first to be open about it. He says his trainers and coaches had never worked with a player with type 1 diabetes before.

"There was a learning curve for pretty much everybody. But the training staff was really cool. They did a lot of research, and they really did everything they could to help me succeed."

Johnson says a low blood sugar incident at spring training early in his minor league career inspired him on his journey to the majors.

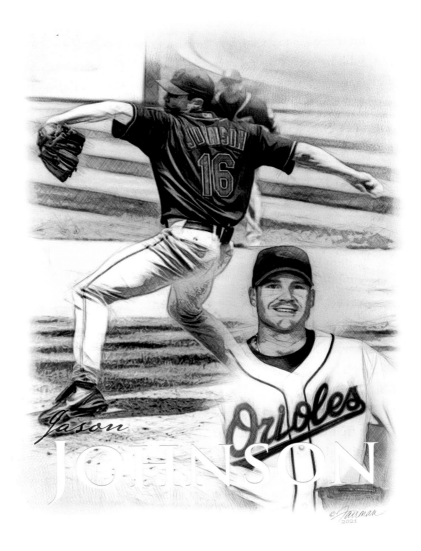

Jason Johnson, American former Major League Baseball pitcher:
"Don't let [diabetes] be the end of you.
Use it is as a building block to make you a better person and a stronger person."

On a hot day of intense workouts at the Pirates minor league camp in Bradenton, Florida, Johnson's blood glucose plummeted and he passed out in the dugout.

"It hit me really fast that day," he says. After some quick nutrition in the clubhouse, he was back to normal. But the Pirates' director of minor leagues panicked, Johnson says, and demanded the young pitcher leave camp to see an endocrinologist before the team would clear him to play again.

"I was like, 'are you serious?'" Johnson says. "'I'm completely fine,'" I told him. "'You know, that happens once in a while when you're diabetic. I promise you, it's not something that's going to happen all the time!'"

The young pitcher continued his protestations while the baseball executive stood firm.

"I was yelling and screaming, telling him it was ridiculous," Johnson laughs. "I called him an idiot. And then I was, immediately, like 'OK, sorry! Didn't mean that.' I was pretty sure I'd get released from the Pirates because I'd just called the director of their minor leagues an idiot. I was like, 'control yourself, Jason!'"

Though he didn't like them, Johnson followed his orders to return home to Kentucky and see his endocrinologist. The physician assured the Pirates that Johnson was fine. The doctor told the Pirates executive that when a person with diabetes exercises as strenuously as professional baseball requires, from time to time that person will experience low blood sugar episodes.

"I missed a week and a half of spring training, but they cleared me to play again."

Johnson says he used that incident as fodder for his determination to make the major leagues.

"I told myself I'd prove to this guy that he was wrong," Johnson says. "I needed to prove that I could be a major league baseball player with diabetes. And I did it."

Johnson says he decided early in his career that he would be as open as possible about having diabetes. He knew he'd encounter teammates and coaches who'd never seen anyone prick his own finger or give himself an injection.

"I just felt it wasn't anything I needed to hide," he says. "I was always straightforward about it. It's funny, I'm still friends with some of the players I met in my first minor league season, back in 1992. I think being open and honest with people leads to friendships like that."

— Expert Commentary —

The decision to share a diagnosis of diabetes with others, especially in the workplace, may be a difficult one to make. You may fear discrimination or getting passed over for opportunities due to your diabetes. Unfortunately, this still sometimes happens in the workplace. This typically occurs when supervisors are unsure about diabetes and how it is treated. If your supervisor is educated about diabetes, they are more likely to understand any unique accommodations you might need to succeed in your job. Consider having an open and frank discussion about your diabetes with your employer. Explain the need to test your glucose regularly, have access to food or beverage at times of a low blood glucose, and signs and symptoms of hypoglycemia. If coworkers and supervisors are well educated on important topics like this, it is less likely diabetes issues impact the work environment. If the director of minor league baseball who was supervising Jason Johnson had understood diabetes and hypoglycemia, the misunderstanding about the response to his low glucose episode could have been avoided.

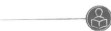

GETTING MIND AND BODY prepared to train or compete is an important part of any athlete's routine. And it's equally important for athletes with diabetes to know when their bodies tell them no.

Since diabetes affects everyone differently and those effects often vary from day to day and even hour to hour, there are times when, no matter how hard the training or how complete the preparations, the athlete needs to take a break. Maybe the break should be for just a few minutes, maybe for a whole game. The self-awareness of knowing when to take a seat on the bench is critical for athletes with diabetes.

It's easy to imagine sitting out a recreation league basketball game or skipping a day of swimming laps because of high or low blood sugar. But what about when the stakes are higher?

As a freshman center at Baylor University, Lauren Cox was still learning the ropes of NCAA women's basketball.

She'd been a star on her high school and her Amateur Athletic Union (AAU) teams, but playing in the Big 12 Conference was another story. Not only is the Big 12 a powerhouse of basketball talent, but games at schools such as Baylor, Iowa State, and Texas are regularly among the best-attended women's games in the country, drawing thousands of fans to their arenas on game nights.

Cox says she was close with her high school and AAU coaches, who understood how to get the most from their 6-foot, 4-inch star despite her diabetes. But stiffer competition, a new coaching staff, and a brighter spotlight were on the horizon for Cox at Baylor.

Cox played in all 37 of her team's games as a freshman, averaging 7.6 points and 4.2 rebounds on a loaded Baylor team that went to the NCAA Tournament's Elite 8, finally losing to eventual tournament runner-up Mississippi State.

By her sophomore season, Cox had adjusted to college and was ready for a bigger role on her team and to display the talent that had made her America's top women's basketball recruit.

In her team's first three games of the 2017–2018 season, Cox started at center and averaged more than 15 points a game. She dom-

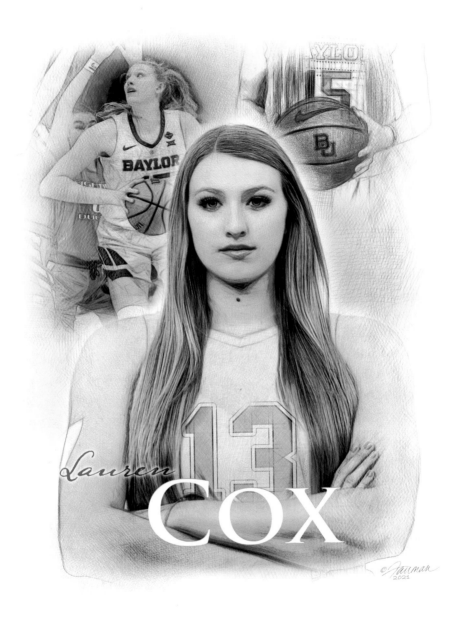

Lauren Cox, American professional basketball player:
"I did everything right . . . it was just one of those days."

inated the last of those games, a Tuesday evening 86–55 home smack-down of an overmatched University of Central Arkansas team. Cox scored 21 points, hauled in 10 rebounds, blocked 2 shots, and even dished out 4 assists in her 33 minutes on the court.

Ranked third in the nation, the Bears looked ready for their next game: a Saturday afternoon, nationally televised game at UCLA's historic Pauley Pavilion against the eighth-ranked Bruins.

But the morning after the Central Arkansas game, Cox could not control her blood sugar. No amount of insulin would lower her glucose.

"It was one of those days," Cox says. "I bolused [insulin] before breakfast, I did everything right. But I just couldn't get my glucose down."

The day after the Central Arkansas game, Cox was dehydrated and nauseated. Team doctors realized that her body needed a lot more insulin than she had on board, sending her blood glucose sky-rocketing and causing her blood to become acidic. She was hospital-ized for diabetic ketoacidosis and would miss the trip to Los Angeles. Without their starting center, Baylor lost at UCLA, 82–68 in a game that was never close.

"I'm a competitor," she says. "I love to be on the court. So that was really frustrating."

Cox recovered from her bout with ketoacidosis quickly. A few days after missing the UCLA game, she traveled with her Baylor teammates to the Bahamas for a Thanksgiving holiday tournament. In games against Missouri State and Georgia Tech, Cox combined for 40 points, 26 rebounds, and 10 blocked shots in lopsided wins for the Bears.

— *Expert Commentary* —

There are bound to be unpredictable situations that arise in the management of a chronic disease such as diabetes. Diabetic ketoacidosis is a medical emer-

gency that can be triggered by an acute event such as an infection, insulin pump malfunction, skipped insulin doses, trauma, surgery, or stressful situations. Following extreme physical exertion, the muscles in the body may sometimes respond to insulin more or less effectively for a few days. It can be frustrating for the patient with diabetes, who may understandably feel a lack of control when these unpredictable situations occur, and it further underscores the importance of having a supportive network when these challenges arise.

PROFESSIONAL CYCLIST Monique Hanley was pretty sure she had her race-day blood sugar regimen just about mastered. Racing in a velodrome—an indoor track with two steep banks and two long straightaways—meant a lot of intense riding, followed by a lot of standing around and waiting for her next race. The Australian had been competing at a high level for a few years and had established her own protocol to manage her diabetes before, during, and after a race.

It could be difficult to predict how long the prerace adrenaline might last, so Hanley kept her blood sugar as low as she could safely keep it.

"After races would start, my blood sugar would increase in the first race and just stay high all night," says Hanley. Were she to aim for normal glucose levels, her adrenaline at the start of the race would shoot her numbers far too high, making her sluggish.

"I'd rather my blood sugar go from about 72 up to 180," she says, "than start it at 145 and then at race time have it at 290 or something."

Before an especially big velodrome race, Hanley says, as she was going through her mental preparations, her coach told her that her first race of the day would be head-to-head against the world champion in women's cycling.

The news was a shock that brought with it a burst of hormones that would affect her blood glucose.

"I didn't anticipate I'd have such a 'fan-girl' moment," she says, laughing.

A cycling fan as much as a cyclist, Hanley had studied the champion and watched her race many times. But she'd never faced her. Hanley became so psyched up for the race that her adrenaline sent her glucose soaring out of control.

"I realized right away that this wasn't a problem I could solve with my little work-around of keeping blood sugar low," she says. "I got so 'up' for the race, that I couldn't get my sugar under control all night."

Her glucose levels made her sluggish for the big race. How'd she do against the champ?

"Terrible," she says. "Sadly, there are no crazy stories about how I beat the world champion with my blood sugar out of control. But I did learn a huge lesson from it."

Disappointed, Hanley says she turned to a sports psychologist for help with a race-day routine. She learned concentration techniques that help her focus and avoid the mental highs and lows that can affect performance.

"I worked a lot on breathing and managing my adrenaline," she says. "My goal is always to make sure diabetes never puts me at a disadvantage. The sports psychologist helped me establish a routine that works for me. That way, no matter what happens, I've still got my routine to keep me calm."

Like most people with diabetes, Hanley's journey hasn't been without occasional difficulty.

On a Monday in 2006, the day after a 150 km race, Hanley was at her office job when she had a seizure. She hadn't recovered sufficiently from the ride; her body didn't yet need the regular dose of insulin it normally needed and her blood glucoses levels dropped.

Interviewed by the *New York Times* about being an athlete with type 1 diabetes, Hanley quipped about a lesson she learned from the diabetic seizure:

"It was a great example of why it would be much better to be a full-time athlete than a full-time office worker."

After her retirement from racing, Hanley established a nonprofit organization in Australia called HypoActive, dedicated to encouraging people with type 1 diabetes to exercise and live active lives.

"The philosophy was basically to help remove barriers to exercise for people with type 1 diabetes," says Hanley. "I didn't need a lot of support in terms of exercise. But what I did need was a social support to keep the mental load of diabetes from becoming too great. That's why I started HypoActive."

— Expert Commentary —

Practical and emotional support is important to feel cared for and one's well-being, especially when living with a chronic disease. For children with diabetes, their parents are the greatest source of influence until adolescence, when friends and peers often become more important as sources of support. In adulthood, a person with diabetes may turn to their spouses or partners, other family members, friends, and colleagues. With adequate social support, the person with diabetes is better able to develop positive coping strategies, deal with stress, engage in good self-management behaviors, and stay motivated. Without it, depression may develop and can lead to greater difficulty in management of diabetes. Organizations such as that founded by Monique Hanley, which include members facing similar challenges, can be incredibly helpful.

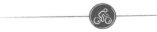

DOMINIQUE WILKINS treats chronic disease like it's an opponent he's determined to beat. Managing his type 2 diabetes is just part of keeping himself healthy, he says.

"I look at having diabetes as a blessing in some ways. It's something that makes me pay attention to what I eat and to moving around, always staying active."

Diagnosed with type 2 about a year after retirement from his hall-of-fame basketball career, Wilkins says the disease hasn't slowed him down. As the NBA's Atlanta Hawks' vice president of basketball and a broadcaster for the team, Wilkins works long days and travels much of the year.

But in addition to staying vigilant about his own health, he's determined to be an advocate for people with diabetes, particularly African Americans.

"When you're in a position to help others who have the same chronic disease as you, I don't think it's really fair not to," he says. "I think we have a responsibility to speak out about it."

"Our community has been devastated by diabetes for years," he says. "My father passed from diabetes. My grandfather had it. I want African Americans to know that it's not a death sentence. It's not a curse. It's an obstacle in the road. It's just something you have to pay attention to until we find a cure for it."

Wilkins has two messages about diabetes for Black Americans: if you don't have it, get screened for it. And if you do have it, take it seriously.

Wilkins says that the toughest part about having diabetes was accepting that he has a chronic disease.

"The most challenging time for me was when I first found out I had it," he says. "I didn't really accept it at first. I think African American men . . . we're very proud. I think sometimes our egos get involved. We might know we have a problem, but we ignore it.

"I'll tell you, though: you can't ignore diabetes. It's not going anywhere. If you find out you have diabetes or prediabetes, you need to accept it and address it. Because if you don't look after it, this disease will catch up to you."

It's perfectly normal to have trouble accepting a diagnosis. After

TABLE 5.2.

Oral and non-insulin injectable medications used in type 2 diabetes

DRUGS BY CLASS	HOW IT WORKS	SOME ADVERSE EFFECTS
Sulfonylureas (oral) *Glyburide* *Glipizide* *Glimepiride*	Stimulates the pancreas to release insulin, which lowers blood glucose	• Risk for low blood glucose • Weight gain
Biguanides (oral) *Metformin*	Reduces insulin resistance in the muscles and reduces liver glucose production	• Nausea, diarrhea, abdominal pain • Vitamin B12 deficiency • Not safe for use with kidney dysfunction
Alpha-glucosidase inhibitors (oral) *Acarbose* *Miglitol*	Slows digestion and absorption of carbohydrates in the gut	• Gas, diarrhea, abdominal pain • Contraindicated with liver or intestinal disease
Meglitinides (oral) *Repaglinide* *Nateglinide*	Stimulate release of insulin just before a meal	• Risk for low blood glucose • Weight gain
Thiazolidinediones (oral) *Pioglitazone* *Rosiglitazone*	Decrease insulin resistance in the muscles, liver, and fat	• Weight gain, edema • Contraindicated in congestive heart failure
DPP-4 inhibitors (oral) *Sitagliptin* *Saxaglipitin* *Linagliptin* *Alogliptin*	Stimulates insulin release with food intake and reduces liver glucose production	• Rare joint pains • Possible pancreatitis
SGLT2 inhibitors (oral) *Canagliflozin* *Empagliflozin* *Dapagliflozin* *Ertugliflozin*	Increases the excretion of glucose by the kidneys into urine	• Increased urination • Acute kidney injury • Increased risk for genital yeast and urinary tract
GLP-1 receptor agonists (mostly injectable; also one oral) *Dulaglutide* *Semaglutide* *Liraglutide* *Lixisenatide* *Exenatide*	Stimulates insulin release with food intake and reduces liver glucose production; decreases appetite and gastric motility	• Nausea, diarrhea, abdominal pain • Contraindicated with prior history of medullary thyroid tumors • Possible pancreatitis

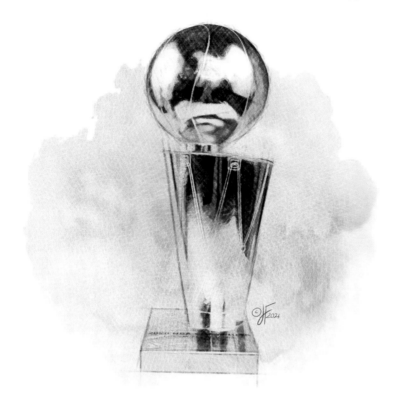

National Basketball Association national championship trophy

Wilkins worked through the stages of acceptance, he says the disease hasn't been too difficult to manage.

"I finally just said to myself, 'OK, this is something in your life that you're going to have to manage and treat the right way.' Twenty years later, I haven't had any problems."

He encourages people to get tested for diabetes. A test called an A1C measures a person's average blood glucose levels over the last three months.

"I treat it very aggressively," he says. "I mean, I never looked at a product label before. I never read the small print to see how much sugar or how many carbs were in something. But I do now."

Wilkins' advocacy work has included participating in a public relations campaign launched by a pharmaceutical company that encourages people with type 2 diabetes to assemble a "diabetes dream team." The concept was for people with the disease to rely on a support system of medical providers, pharmacists, family members, and others who can help lessen the burden.

"You don't have to do it by yourself," he says. "That's important to remember. The people who care about you can help."

He says his family is well-versed in the details of diabetes management.

"They don't have a choice," he says, laughing. "Because I'm so heavily involved with it, they hear me talk about it all the time."

— *Expert Commentary* —

Racial and ethnic minorities such as African Americans, Asians, Hispanics, and Pacific Islanders are much more likely than others to develop type 2 diabetes, which represents 90%–95% of all diabetes cases. Persons with type 2 diabetes are more "resistant" to the effects of insulin; in other words, the insulin produced by their body is not as effective at lowering blood glucose. Type 2 diabetes can initially be treated with oral medications that either improve the ability of the body to respond to insulin, stimulate the body to produce more insulin, reduce carbohydrate absorption in the gut, or increase glucose excretion by the kidneys into urine (Table 5.2). There are also non-insulin injections, also known as GLP-1 receptor agonists, that are given daily or weekly and can lead to moderate weight loss in type 2 diabetes. Over time, insulin injections may sometimes be required as part of the natural progression of the disease. Community education is especially important in encouraging high-risk individuals to be screened for prediabetes and type 2 diabetes so that diabetes can be diagnosed in a timely manner. Approximately 1 in 5 individuals with diabetes remain undiagnosed and don't even know that they have the disease. The support of family and friends can help the patient with newly diagnosed diabetes take their disease seriously and seek out the appropriate treatment. All people with diabetes should have the benefit of a "diabetes dream team" that can help them feel less isolated and ensure that they thrive while living with diabetes.

MISSY FOY was ready to make history.

The North Carolina marathoner had traveled to Columbia, South Carolina, for a race that could qualify her to compete in the 2000 Summer Olympic Games in Sydney, Australia.

Considered a long shot for the Olympic team, Foy was thrilled to be among only 170 runners to be invited to the trials race. But the night before the race, event officials sent a note to Foy's hotel room telling her that she was disqualified from the race because she used a substance that was banned by the International Olympic Committee: insulin.

Insulin is an anabolic hormone, which means that it builds and promotes storage of carbohydrates, fats, and proteins in the body. Some athletes have misused insulin as a way to build muscle mass, similar to the way they use anabolic steroids.

After Foy protested to race officials that she had diabetes, the organizers sent a local physician to confirm that her use of insulin wasn't meant to cheat her fellow competitors; she needed it to survive.

The physician confirmed that Foy did, in fact, have type 1 diabetes. She was cleared to compete only hours before the starting gun. Foy finished the Olympic Trial marathon in under three hours, placing her in the middle of the pack. Because of unusually hot conditions that day, only one runner qualified for the Olympic team.

Foy was—and remains—the only marathoner with diabetes to compete for a spot on the Olympic team, having twice qualified for the Olympic Trials.

When Foy took up running in her early 30s, it came far easier to her than to most people. Within a few months of deciding to compete, she began not just finishing races but winning them. In February 1997, she won the women's national championship for 8 km racing.

But in August of that same year, having just qualified for the national championship for half marathon, she was diagnosed with type 1 diabetes. A case of food poisoning sent her to the emergency room. After some blood tests, intravenous fluids, and anti-nausea medicine, an emergency physician asked her if she had any family history of diabetes.

"No. Why?"

"Your blood glucose reading is high."

"Really? How high?"

"860."

Healthy blood glucose for adults should be under 100 milligrams per deciliter of blood. Foy's was eight times too high. She felt certain there had been a lab error in reading her test.

"Yeah, you're probably right," the emergency physician said.

But when they tested her again, Foy says the device the hospital uses to measure blood glucose read only "High." Her sugar was too high to even measure.

Crushed when she got her diagnosis, Foy was convinced her burgeoning running career was over.

"I cried for days after that," she says.

But little by little, she inched back to the idea that she could continue competing. She would, of course, need a good endocrinologist who supported her competitive running and who would work with her to find ways to manage diabetes.

The search proved difficult. Four different endocrinologists told her they couldn't imagine competing at an elite level with type 1 diabetes. Foy adjusted her search to include a physician who specialized in both diabetes and sports medicine.

She found one at a regional academic medical center about 60 miles from her home. Foy emailed the doctor and asked if he could help her. A runner himself, he told Foy he understood her situation. Recalling their electronic correspondence, she says he was less than encouraging.

"He just didn't even think it was a possibility. He wrote me something like, 'from one runner to another, if someone with diabetes could run Olympic marathons, it already would've been done.'"

Foy decided she'd have to learn how to manage her diabetes herself. Later that year, she ran a marathon that qualified her to compete in the Olympic Trials. The first person she emailed after the race was the diabetes and sports medicine physician.

"I hit 'reply' and I only wrote one sentence," she says. "I wrote, 'It's been done.'"

For years, Foy trained at Duke University's athletic complex, alongside the school's student–athletes. Foy learned of her near superhuman ability to use oxygen during exercise at a research center on campus. The VO2 max measures the maximum rate of oxygen a person can absorb and use during strenuous physical exertion. An excellent female athlete can expect a VO2 max between about 31 and 36. Foy's maximum?

"It's kind of freaky," she says, sheepishly. "It's 74."

Discovering that her capacity to use oxygen during exercise is more than twice as great as many of the world's greatest women athletes meant that Foy is built for endurance running.

As a result, in 2005, she began competing in long-distance races known as ultramarathons. Foy won the first such race she ever ran, a 50-mile event held near her North Carolina home. She finished the race in 7 hours, 15 minutes, and 6 seconds, smashing the course record by 20 minutes.

Foy earned a top-10 world ranking in 50-mile racing in 2005 and finished second in the US 50-Mile National Championships in 2007.

In addition to being an elite athlete, Foy is an academic. Part of her program to earn a PhD in the history of medicine was to complete many of the same classes that medical students typically take. She understands her own physiology better than most people. For instance, she says her old glucose management routine probably didn't do her many favors.

"I look back now and I think it was probably a mistake to let my blood sugar go low during training or during a race," she says.

While some athletes who have diabetes have said their strategy is to let their blood sugar dip to the lower end of normal before a competition, Foy believes that extreme exertion regularly depleted the glycogen reserves in her muscles, blood, and liver. Glycogen is the storage form of glucose in the body.

"It was all gone," she says. Letting her fuel tank go completely empty, so to speak, depleted her of an important energy source: glucose.

After that discovery, Foy began using small office-supply binder clips to attach 1-ounce packets of energy gel to her shorts and shirt during training and races. The gel is packed full of easy-to-digest carbohydrates that keep Foy's muscles fueled. Without breaking stride, she unclips a packet, bites off the top, and squeezes the concentrated contents into her mouth. In minutes, her system begins to convert the carbohydrates to energy, allowing Foy to keep pushing toward the tape.

Other mid-race nutrition includes peanut butter and jelly sandwiches.

"I can eat while I run, sandwich in one hand, water in the other. It takes me about a mile to get it down without throwing it back up. It took a little practice to master." Foy also drinks water at every water station on the course.

"Staying hydrated is absolutely key," she says. "If you dehydrate, you're going to get nauseated and you can't take nourishment. When that happens, that's the end of your race."

As Foy gained more success as a runner, her competitors became

When Kylee Perez's father would test her blood sugar through the chain-link fence at a softball game, he was also sending her the message that diabetes is nothing to be ashamed of. It's not weird or creepy. It doesn't make a person different.

Dominique Wilkins was retired from basketball when he learned he has diabetes. He could easily have kept it quiet, managing the disease on his own, keeping it private. But he chose to be a spokesperson and role model for others, especially Black Americans.

Perez, Wilkins, and the others in this chapter and book set the example that diabetes doesn't define them. It's just a chronic disease that needs attention.

Chapter 6

Winning with Diabetes
Can I accomplish my life goals?

"DIABETES HASN'T held me back at all," says Baltimore Ravens All-Pro tight end Mark Andrews. "Quite the opposite. Putting a high priority on sports means you put a high priority on your health. I've been able to take care of my body and learn my body in a way that most people don't have to—even other professional athletes. That's allowed me to play at the highest levels."

Drafted in the third round by the Ravens, Andrews made an impact in the NFL right away. He set a Ravens rookie record for catches and receiving yards, emerging as a favorite receiver of 2018 quarterbacks Joe Flacco and Lamar Jackson. In 2019, his second season in the NFL, Andrews was named to the AFC Pro Bowl team after catching 64 passes, 10 of which were for touchdowns and 44 of which gained his team a first down. In 2020, Andrews helped the Ravens get off to a hot start, catching two touchdown passes in the season opener against Cleveland and two more a few weeks later against Washington.

The Scottsdale, Arizona, native earned unanimous All-American honors in his junior season at the University of Oklahoma, winning

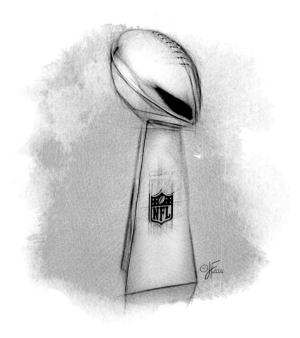

National Football League Super Bowl championship trophy

the John Mackey Award as college football's most outstanding tight end. He declared himself eligible for the NFL draft following that season.

Mark Andrews's physician father continues to be intimately involved with his son's game-day diabetes management.

"I don't really like to bug [the Ravens'] training staff with my blood sugar numbers" during games, Andrews said. "So, I have my mom and dad and my brother connected on my monitor."

"Oh, and my agent too."

Even with his family and representation keeping an eye on his blood sugar, Andrews knows he's in charge of his own health.

"Seventy-five percent of my normal basal rate is through a long-acting insulin [injection]," Andrews explained of his routine on days when he's practicing with the Ravens. "And the other 25% comes from my pump."

Game days are different.

"I like to go 100% on long-acting insulin [injection] just because I'm off the pump for so many hours at a time. That gives me the freedom to not really worry about my numbers fluctuating too much."

Andrews said he's heard of some football players with diabetes who make space for a pump under their protective pads. But taking a hit from a defender while wearing an insulin pump doesn't appeal to him.

"Personally, I just feel freer without one. I'm able to do what I have to do without thinking about it."

He admits to a game-day secret weapon: peanut butter.

"That's my big complex carb source before and during the game," he said. "The night before and then a couple hours before the game, I eat a ton of peanut butter and jelly sandwiches.

"I love peanut butter."

His diet is working: Andrews said he's never missed a down because of his diabetes.

"I don't let the numbers go too high or too low during a game. [Football] is my job now, so there's more at stake. But it's always been incredibly important to me not to let diabetes affect my game."

Andrews didn't always line up next to an offensive tackle. As a standout at Scottsdale Desert Mountain High School, Andrews was a sure-handed wide receiver, amassing nearly 3,700 yards receiving and 48 touchdowns in three seasons.

But because he was a shade slower than average for a wide receiver in the NCAA's Big 12 Conference, the Sooners envisioned the 6-foot 5-inch Andrews as a tight end. While wide receivers are typically asked to block similarly sized defensive backs, tight ends frequently engage with bigger and stronger linemen and linebackers.

So, Andrews's Oklahoma coaches asked him to put on some weight. At 225 pounds, they told him, he could catch passes, but he wasn't bulky or strong enough to do the physical dirty work often asked of tight ends.

Andrews agreed with the decision and redshirted during his first year at Oklahoma, concentrating on getting big enough to play his new position.

"I kind of saw the writing on the wall," he said. "I was going to need to put on weight."

But if not done properly, weight gain can cause problems for people with diabetes. Like many Division I football programs, Oklahoma has nutritionists on staff. Andrews credits Tiffany Byrd, the Sooners' director of sports nutrition, with helping him bulk up without throwing his blood sugar into a spin.

"We called her Coach T," Andrews recalled, adding that OU's nutritionists enjoy rare status among the team and football staff. Byrd worked closely with Andrews, designing a special muscle-building program with his diabetes in mind.

"Usually, guys take high-protein, high-carbs right after [a weight-lifting session]. That wasn't something I wanted to do," he said.

Andrews needed to avoid foods or drinks that would send his blood sugar too high.

"Coach T and I were able to work out something where after lifting, I'd have a shake that was made from whey protein."

A concoction high in protein but low in carbohydrates would feed his muscles after an intense workout, but it wouldn't drop a dangerous "carb bomb" on his system.

"That way, I could get the fuel I needed and gain weight, but not gain the bad weight."

By the time he played his first down at Oklahoma in 2015, Andrews was 31 muscular pounds heavier than he'd been in high school.

Understanding what his body needs and how those needs might differ from teammates has been a hallmark of Andrews's football career; he's always known he has to be aware of his diabetes at all times.

BOX 6.1
Diabetes and Exercise

Not all exercise is equal with regard to the effect on blood glucose in patients with diabetes. The use of continuous glucose monitors has substantially improved our understanding of how patients with diabetes respond to exercise and can allow you to help keep glucose levels in a desired range before and after exercise. Here are some basic principles to consider regarding exercise:

1. Regardless of exercise type or duration, the ultimate endpoint leads to a lower glucose. It may not occur right away, but ultimately, exercise lowers glucose due to increased uptake of glucose into skeletal muscle. Rarely, blood glucoses can spike after certain resistance or muscle-strengthening exercises if insulin becomes less effective for a short period of time (insulin resistance).

2. Interval training is a special circumstance that can lead to an initial rise in blood glucose and then followed by glucose levels falling. For aerobic exercise this may look like running one lap as fast as you can on a track followed by two really slow laps and then repeating the cycle. With the one really fast lap, your glucose may rise. With the two really slow laps, your glucose may fall. This pattern can continue to repeat during the workout. For resistance training, this may look like lifting heavy weights with low repetitions. The weightlifter may see an initial burst in glucose levels, followed by levels falling in between sets of exercise.

3. Low-intensity training typically leads to a slow and steady reduction of glucose during the workout. For aerobic exercise, this may look like running moderate-intensity laps continuously around a track. For resistance training, this would involve lighter weights with higher repetitions.

4. Stress hormones surrounding the training may also play a role in glucose levels. "Butterflies" in your stomach that an athlete might feel before a big game come from a rise in stress hormones such as epinephrine (adrenaline), growth hormone, or cortisol; subsequently, this can result in a sharp, brief rise in glucose values.

5. Practice makes perfect—with blood glucose control during exercise as well. Everyone responds slightly differently to exercise. Reviewing your plan for exercise, evaluating the response of your glucose during and after the activity, discussing results with your diabetes provider, and then making adjustments regularly as needed can work well.

During intense workouts and practices, whether at Oklahoma or with the Ravens, Andrews pays close attention to his own body's signals. He's not afraid to step away if he needs to.

"No one gets to this level without being a competitive person by nature," Andrews explained. "But there's a certain maturity that I gained at a very young age and I know that, with diabetes, there are going to be days where I feel more tired than I should."

Those days are when, Andrews said, he steps aside, checks his blood sugar, and does what he needs to do to get back in balance.

"Maybe those days, I'm not as hydrated as I should be," he said. "I'm losing everything quicker than everybody else and I need to stop. I'm lucky that I've never been pressured into situations I shouldn't be in."

Besides peanut butter, Andrews said his formula for successful management of his diabetes comes down to two ingredients. The first: vigilance.

"If you've got diabetes, it's 24/7," he said. "Even when you're sleeping, it's not something you can forget about. The minute you do, it's going to bite you."

The second ingredient: good people.

"Surround yourself with people who care about you," he advises. "There'll definitely be some complications along the way with diabetes, but if you know yourself and you have those people to help look after you, everything is good."

Andrews said he's never had a teammate or coach with diabetes. He's always been open to explaining the disease to his peers. He recalled a scene in the locker room before a Ravens preseason game, where teammates saw him testing his blood sugar about two hours before kickoff.

"A bunch of my tight end buddies came over and they all asked me to test them too," he laughed. He changed the lancet for five different players and tested each of their sugars.

"I was able to kind of show them a little bit of what my life is like," he said.

— *Expert Commentary* —

Exercise definitely has effects on blood glucose (Box 6.1). This holds true for a walk in your neighborhood, a session in the gym, or an NFL game. If you use an insulin pump, you have some choices to make with what to do with your pump during physical activity. There are multiple factors to consider, and discussing these options with your diabetes provider is a good idea.

- *Will the workout be short or long?*
- *Will the intensity be high or low?*
- *Will the type of exercise be aerobic or resistance?*
- *Is there physical contact involved in the activity?*

Mark Andrews removes his pump on game days and instead uses a long-acting basal insulin injection. He does this because of the lack of practicality of wearing his pump while being tackled by 250-pound linebackers and the need to have the pump off for a long time during game day. If Andrews was participating in a shorter duration noncontact sport where the game or competition only lasted about 60 minutes or less, he may choose to just take off his pump for that hour and go without insulin for that time. This can be safe for up to approximately two hours in consultation with the physician, but it can get tricky for durations longer than this. Another option an insulin pump user could consider is the use of an "exercise mode." Integrated insulin pumps and glucose sensors take information from the glucose sensor to help the pump deliver the correct amount of insulin to achieve a certain glucose target. These integrated pumps and sensors have "exercise" settings that tell the pump's algorithm to target a higher glucose level to help minimize hypoglycemia during and after exercise.

AT 29, JASON JOHNSON had pitched parts of seven seasons in the major leagues. He was used to his between-innings ritual of testing his blood sugar and doing what he needed to do to avoid highs or lows.

But in 2003, he discovered that an insulin pump made managing his type 1 diabetes a lot easier. He still paid close attention to his glucose levels, but he was able to leave the finger sticks and test strips behind.

Except for when he pitched.

"It never even occurred to me to wear it on the pitcher's mound," he says now.

It wasn't until the next season, as a veteran, free-agent starter for the Detroit Tigers, that Johnson asked Major League Baseball to allow him to be the first big leaguer to wear an insulin pump on the field.

"Our trainer, Kevin Rand, convinced me to try it," says Johnson.

Before the pump, Johnson's pregame rituals included making sure his blood sugar was somewhere between 150 and 160 md/dl. He understood that the physical and mental demands of pitching in a major league game would cause that number to fall relatively quickly.

"Any higher than that, I didn't feel good," he says. High glucose numbers meant that Johnson felt sluggish and tired, he says. "But I knew if I started the game at around 150, I'd be good through about three innings. After that, I'd drink a Gatorade to get my sugar back up."

Johnson earned a reputation around the big leagues as a durable starter who could keep his team in games for six or seven innings. His diabetes didn't affect his 11-year major league career, where he pitched for eight different teams. Johnson's longest stints were five seasons in Baltimore and two in Detroit.

Johnson says that, before the pump, he went through about six glucose test strips a game. After pitching an inning, he'd stick his finger for a blood test. While it wasn't common for him to need a shot of insulin during a game, he says it did happen.

"I didn't have to do that a lot," he recalls. "Probably four or five times."

While normally, physical exertion would make his sugar drop, on those occasions his tests told Johnson his glucose was near 200 mg/dl.

"I can't pitch like that. So, I would run back into the clubhouse in between innings and pray that our hitters didn't make three quick outs. I'd fill a shot needle with insulin really quick and get back out there."

Similarly, when Johnson felt his sugar drop, he hoped for long innings while his team was at bat. As soon as he returned to the dugout, he'd check his sugar.

"If it got down to 50 or 60 mg/dl" and his team's batters made quick outs, "I was like, 'oh man, I'm in trouble,'" he says. "I'd eat and drink as fast as I could before I went back out to the mound."

One day in the spring of 2004, the Tigers trainer asked Johnson if he'd considered wearing his insulin pump when he pitched.

"I never had. I'd wear the pump all day, then right before the game I'd disconnect it," he says. "I'd keep it in my locker and then I'd have to check my sugar between innings again."

But when Rand brought it up, Johnson agreed it was time to petition the league to let him wear a pump.

"They told us they'd make a decision in two or three weeks," Johnson remembers. "But it only took them three days. Major League Baseball was great about it."

Being the first major league baseball player with diabetes to use an insulin pump while playing against the best baseball players in the world meant Johnson needed to experiment with infusion sites and the best place to attach the pump to his Tigers uniform.

He knew he had to wear the pump in a spot where it was safe from line drives. He also knew he had to insert the infusion needle under the skin on a spot on where it wouldn't get yanked out by the extreme torque that a major league pitcher generates during his delivery.

Johnson decided to clip the pump to his belt near the small of his back, a few inches below his uniform number.

The infusion site was another matter. The small tube that leads from the infusion site to the pump needed to remain secure.

Throughout his career, Johnson was primarily a low 90s fastball pitcher, mixing in some off-speed and breaking pitches to keep hitters off balance. At 6 feet, 6 inches tall and a playing weight of about 215 pounds, Johnson relied on his body's motion to generate the power behind his pitches.

"I had a few issues early in that season where the infusion set ripped out" and ruined the pump, recalls Johnson. "I remember thinking, when it happened, 'Aw man! Those things aren't cheap!'"

The combination of sweat and Johnson's kinetic windup made it hard to keep his infusion set taped to his body and attached to the pump. After some experimenting, he found a better area to infuse—a spot on the back of one of his hips—and the right way to stick the tube to his skin. The tape that came with the pump wasn't designed for athletic activity, let alone Major League Baseball. So, Johnson found a waterproof tape used in hospitals.

"I didn't have any issues after that."

Johnson was Detroit's Opening Day starter against the Blue Jays that season. Wearing an insulin pump on the mound for the first time in his career, Johnson pitched six scoreless innings in Toronto's SkyDome (now known as the Rogers Centre), earning the win against future Hall of Famer Roy Halladay.

While his team finished the 2004 season in a distant fourth place in the American League Central, Johnson posted career highs in starts (33) and innings pitched (1962⁄3), including a complete-game, 11-strikeout shutout in Minnesota in July. The pump was a success.

— Expert Commentary —

The problems Jason Johnson faced with where to place his pump and keeping it in place are not unique. Every insulin pump user faces decisions about where to place their pump infusion site and/or continuous glucose monitor repeatedly over time. Following some basic principles can help make diabetes technologies easier to use in the long term.

The first basic principle is "rotation, rotation, rotation." The pump infusion site needs to be regularly rotated to prevent scarring and lipohypertrophy, which is a lump under the skin caused by accumulation of extra fat at the site of insulin infusion. This can also occur with injections of subcutaneous injections of insulin in type 1 or type 2 diabetes. If the injection sites are not rotated routinely, these scarring changes will lead to uneven insulin absorption and high blood glucose.

Traditionally, pump infusion sites can be placed in the abdomen below the rib cage as long as they are 2 inches or more away from the umbilicus (belly button). When picking a new site, you should move a few inches away from the prior site. Aside from the abdomen, some people place their infusion sites on the upper buttocks, low back ("love handle" area), or upper legs. Sites should be changed at least every three days. If you are infusing large amounts of insulin through your pump, you may need to change the site more often (every two days) to allow consistent absorption. This is also true for individuals who use insulin injections.

Continuous glucose monitor sites are dependent on the type of sensor. Some are approved for the abdomen and some for the back of the upper arm. These sites are changed anywhere from 7 to 14 days depending on the model being used. Allergic reactions do sometimes occur in relation to the adhesive from the sensor or the insulin infusion site. Steroid sprays applied to the skin before applying the device can help blunt these reactions. Sometimes barrier patches or specialized bandages can be applied to the skin and then the sensor applied through this. The barrier works by placing a layer between the skin and the adhesive that is causing the reaction.

A TRACK AND FIELD MEET can be an all-day affair. In addition to multiple events that involve jumping or throwing, there are various sprints and longer-distance races, hurdles, and relays. There are men's and women's competitions and often several different age categories in which to compete.

Though Kate Hall-Harnden focuses mainly on the long jump now, she occasionally competes in the 60-meter sprint, a non-Olympic event held mostly indoors. Since that race is a dash of a little under 200 feet, the event itself is finished in less than 10 seconds. That makes keeping blood sugar at optimum competition levels relatively simple.

But for a long jump event alone, there can be a dozen or more competitors attempting multiple jumps, with delays of several minutes between each jump. Like all elite athletes, the jumpers must maintain sharp mental focus and loose muscles between jumps. Keeping her blood sugar at a consistent level throughout the long jump event is crucial for Hall-Harnden.

"The whole long jump event can last an hour or an hour and a half," says Hall-Harnden. "And because I'm so competitive, I have a lot of adrenaline while it's happening."

"My blood sugar is good at the beginning, but then as I start jumping, it spikes really, really fast. And there still might be another hour to go," Hall-Harnden says. "It's hard. Because I want to focus on the competition and not always be checking my blood sugar. But I also don't want it to spike to, like, 300 mg/dl or something."

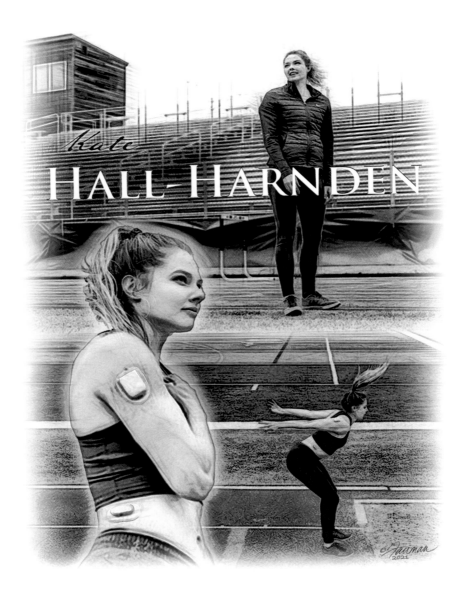

Kate Hall-Harnden, American track and field athlete
and national high school record holder in the long jump and
NCAA champion who previously qualified for the final
at the United States Olympic Trials:
*"[Diabetes] is just something I'm still trying to learn more about
and figure out a way of dealing with."*

The long jump requires near-perfect technique and muscle memory. Often, only a few inches separate the winner from the bottom finishers. At Hall-Harnden's level of competition, jumpers take between 20 and 22 strides in their runway approach, building speed gradually and using the last two strides to set up an optimum launch angle at the greatest possible momentum. Jumpers' feet must be positioned perfectly at the takeoff and then, in midair, the athlete repositions her body's center of gravity using her arms and legs. Then, landing in a sandpit, the jumper needs to make sure her bottom doesn't touch the sand between her heels and the jump-off point, which would cost her precious inches in her jump's measurement.

"It's so technical and everything has to be perfect," Hall-Harnden says.

She experiments to find the optimum glucose range for starting an event.

"For a long time, I started at around 150 mg/dl," she explains. "And I never know how high it's going to get. It depends on the competition." At important meets, she says, her blood sugar can zoom as high as 300 md/dl.

"I'm trying to start it a little lower, so it won't spike quite so high," she says. "That's something I'm still working on."

Anyone who has ever competed in anything knows that practice and game-day competition are completely different. But for people with diabetes, they're even more different. While Hall-Harnden's glucose numbers are high on days when she's competing at a track and field meet, the opposite is true for practice days.

"My sugar would always go really low during training," she says. "I didn't really know how to deal with that at first. So, I would just have a juice box or something. And then my blood sugar would go really high. It was like a roller coaster."

"It's just something I'm still trying to learn more about and figure out a way of dealing with it."

— Expert Commentary —

Kate Hall-Harnden notes that her glucose levels sometimes go really low during her training and then she has to correct them with juice, which then spikes her levels too high, leading to a "roller coaster" effect. This is a common problem for patients with diabetes. In contrast, the A1C blood test is a commonly used marker of long-term glucose levels and reflects the average of glucose numbers over the prior 90 to 120 days. Simply put, a lower A1C means a lower glucose average and a higher A1C means a higher glucose average. But the story is not that simple.

Using insulin, we can achieve a low glucose average in almost any person but, if this is at the expense of a roller coaster of glucose extremes, it might not be a good thing. Diabetes care focus has moved beyond just the A1C to now additionally consider things like "time in range" and "standard deviation or glucose variability." These are statistical measurements that can be found when reviewing data from continuous glucose monitors. TIR (time in range) is the percentage of glucose readings between the target range of 70 and 180 md/dl. SD (standard deviation) and GV (glucose variability) are measures of how high and low glucose values rise and fall throughout the day. The goal is a high TIR and a low SD. Individual goals vary for patients but, in general, aiming for >70% TIR is appropriate for otherwise healthy patients with diabetes. Maintaining a high time in range with a low glucose variability reduces dangerous hypoglycemia and minimizes problems of fatigue and a lack of focus that can occur. Achieving these diabetes goals helps an elite athlete like Kate Hall-Harnden achieve her athletic goals and also can help non-athletes in the home, workplace, and daily life.

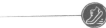

When a person is introduced with the words "despite having type 1 diabetes . . . ," it seems as likely as not that the introduction will be of Will Cross.

In 2001, as a 34-year-old teacher in Pittsburgh's northern suburbs, Cross began an extraordinary journey to raise money for diabetes research and to prove that the disease doesn't have to slow anyone
down. First stop: the North Pole.

Cross convinced a company that manufactures medical supplies
for people with diabetes to sponsor his treks to the top and bottom
of the earth. In addition to raising publicity and awareness of type 1
diabetes, the journeys to the North and South Poles could provide
valuable insight into whether people with the disease should be lim-
ited in their pursuits of this kind of adventure. They hoped to answer
questions about the durability and effectiveness of glucose-testing
equipment and insulin in extreme conditions. And they wondered
whether the increased blue light that exists at the earth's poles—
which comes from sunlight reflecting off bright white frozen surfaces—would damage the eyes of people who have diabetes, particularly those that have decreased blood perfusion of blood vessels in the
retina.

The earth's axis at the top of the globe is about 700 miles from the
nearest land. There are no bridges or roads or airports at the North
Pole. There's no sign or visitors center. Only ice and blue ocean, more
than two and half miles deep.

The constantly shifting ice floes in the Arctic Ocean are between
6 and 10 feet thick. Rather than a smooth surface like a skating rink,
the ice at the pole is rough and dangerous. Powerful slow-motion
collisions of miles-wide drifts form icy hills as tall as 200 feet and ob-
stacles that are often unstable and a challenge to navigate.

In April, Cross and a fellow trekker flew from Pittsburgh to a tiny
island a few hundred miles off the coast of Norway. A helicopter then
dropped them off at the edge of a permanent ice pack, about 100
miles from the North Pole.

The month of April offers the best hiking weather in the Arctic.
The sun doesn't set and temperatures are near −20°F.

Constantly shifting ice means there are no maps of the most efficient route across the surface. Pushing and dragging heavy sleds full of supplies, Cross and his companion encountered numerous dead ends that required backtracking and trying another approach. Often, at the end of a long day of hiking, they made camp at the edge of a great ice drift in hopes that it would freeze to an adjacent frozen slab. If it did, they'd walk across in the direction of the pole. If it didn't, they'd turn around, retrace their steps, and find new ice to hike. Sometimes they strapped on cross-country skis and sloshed their way forward.

The pair pulled 100-pound sleds full of supplies over the frozen Arctic, avoiding the frigid, churning waters beneath the shifting ice. Averaging about 10 hours of walking a day, Cross survived the journey on a daily 6,000-calorie diet that included chocolate bars and cheese, among other high-fat foods.

In addition to food, water, tents, sleeping bags, and tools, Cross had to pack several weeks' worth of insulin for the long, frozen-ocean walk.

Cross calls his walk to the North Pole "a short trip," at about two weeks. Among the things he needed to find out were how to best protect his insulin from the elements, what kind of diet to eat, and whether the increased blue light at the top and bottom of the earth would affect his vision.

On April 20, 2000, Will Cross became the first person with diabetes to walk to the North Pole. And he was just getting warmed up. Cross says his walk to the very top of the earth prepared him for the more-difficult trek at the bottom, two years later.

Because it's in the middle of a land mass and sits under a 900-foot-thick block of ice, the South Pole's conditions are far harsher than those at the North Pole. And it was a much longer journey.

A few years later, Cross walked across more than 700 miles to the South Pole. He has summited Mount Everest and other Nepalese peaks several times.

Climbing the world's tallest mountains and crossing its harshest landscapes isn't just difficult. It's also expensive.

Training, transportation, Sherpas, oxygen, and supplies aren't cheap. And then there are the permits: to climb Mount Everest from its south side requires a costly permit from the Tibet Tourism Bureau. In all, it's common for the journey to the top of the world to cost $60,000 to $70,000.

Athletes who want to take on extreme challenges like the ones Will Cross has completed regularly solicit sponsorship for their excursions from big companies hoping to align themselves with the adventure, dedication, and wonder that comes with big endeavors. In exchange for promotion and media exposure, the companies finance some—or even all—of the trek.

Will Cross hadn't yet climbed Mount Everest. So, his proposal to potential sponsors of his trek across the coldest, most remote place on earth was met with some skepticism. The 35-year-old Cross wanted to walk the 730 miles across Antarctica to the South Pole.

The South Pole is a frozen desert, which means it doesn't get much snow—less than half an inch a year. But the snow it does get never melts. Thus, the surface is a giant chunk of ice that's almost two miles above sea level.

It's tempting to envision the desolate, unspoiled South Pole as a pristine sheet of clear ice, like some kind of never-used skating rink. But in reality, the surface of the ice is rough, craggy, and dangerous. And if that weren't enough, the 9,300-foot altitude makes crossing the South Pole even more difficult and treacherous.

Cross told his sponsors the 730-mile journey would take two months. He and a traveling partner would pile their supplies onto long sleds with sharp steel runners. They would drag the heaps across the bumpy, frozen surface.

"The sponsors told me they weren't sure that I could last 60 days pulling a 200-pound sled" in one of the coldest climates on earth.

"They thought I would get frostbite and lose a hand or a foot. Or that I'd go blind from the bright light at the South Pole."

Because of its white surface, the South Pole reflects nearly all the ultraviolet light the sun shines on it, creating a blinding effect. Because diabetes can cause retinal damage, Cross says his potential funders worried the light would further complicate Cross's hike.

"Sponsors and investors want to make sure they're not supporting a death march," he says. "They don't want anyone getting injured or stuck out there. I knew I could do it, but I didn't have any data to prove it."

So, with help from some physiology scientists at the University of Pittsburgh, Cross set out to convince his sponsors he could survive the journey and to prove that he knew how to avoid the dangers that a person with diabetes would face.

"For example, cuts take longer to heal because the endocrine system is compromised. Just a simple cut or a mild case of frostbite could turn septic and get dangerous really quickly," says Cross. "So, we did a lot of testing to prove that I knew how to manage that risk."

He included in his sponsorship proposals that he'd follow a diet that many Norwegians eat in extreme cold.

"It's about 50% fat. That's the best way to get the most calories while still keeping things small enough to carry."

To fuel the journey, Cross would need to consume about 6,000 calories each day. Thick soups and stews, lots of nuts, energy drinks, sugary hydration drinks, chocolate, and calorie-heavy pudding would become dietary staples.

What's more, in the months before he even left his home town of Pittsburgh, Cross packed on 30 pounds of fat. He ate high-fat foods that people with diabetes should be careful with. Potato chips, ice cream, junk food—all of it was meant to provide a store of reserve energy for the grueling journey of 10-hour days, pulling his sled full of supplies in temperatures that regularly reached –30°F.

Even as he plumped up for the trip, Cross trained hard, biking and working out on stair-climber and rowing machines.

He says the sponsors needed to be convinced that a diet so high in fat wouldn't send his cholesterol soaring and cause a heart attack or stroke. Allaying sponsor fears one by one, Cross, along with the Pitt physiologists, proved he was as capable as anyone to endure the journey.

The things that worried sponsors didn't trouble Cross. He'd proven his physical and mental capabilities and was confident he was ready to take on the South Pole.

But one question stuck with him: what if he needed to be rescued? If he got injured or if a severe storm made crossing Antarctica impossible, Cross figured that, in bad weather conditions, it could take a rescue team as long as five days to reach him.

And if storms at the South Pole got bad enough that Cross needed to be rescued, he figured it was also possible his supply of insulin might freeze. He wouldn't survive five days waiting to be rescued without insulin.

Drug manufacturers universally warn against exposing insulin to extreme temperatures. Freezing insulin causes changes in the hormone's molecular structure, making it less effective. It is also usually recommended to discard insulin that has been frozen. But Cross experimented and put a vial in his kitchen freezer. After it thawed, he injected a dose.

"I mean, it wasn't great," he says. "I'd say it was about 30% effective."

Still, Cross calculated that, while by no means ideal, he could survive on the once-frozen insulin until a rescue team reached him.

His sponsors finally convinced, in October 2002 Cross and his traveling partner set off for the South Pole. Harnessed ahead of their sleds by their waists and shoulders, they crossed the frozen bottom of the earth.

In the mornings, Cross's first glucose reading was regularly around 100 mg/dl. His breakfast boosted him to about 220 to get his day started. But as he and his partner steadily put one ski in front the other, his sugar descended to more normal ranges.

Days began at 6:30 a.m., with a calorie-packed breakfast and a pot of coffee that also contained a huge plop of powdered butter. Cross and his partner aimed to walk about 13 miles each day. They'd power ahead for 90-minute stretches, eating nuts and chocolate all the while. Ten-minute breaks were for even more eating.

They set up camp each night around 7:00 p.m., after a big dinner and a satellite-phone call home. They also kept various media outlets apprised of their progress.

Day-to-day recovery posed the greatest challenge of the trip, says Cross.

"Our bodies don't recover as quickly" as people without diabetes, he says. "Punishing yourself 10 hours a day for two months" would be tough for any athlete. But bouncing back, day after day, was the hardest part, according to Cross.

Another challenge: testing blood glucose in temperatures far below zero, with polar winds whipping. Cross says he could only test his sugar when he was cocooned in his sleeping bag inside his tent. That meant only two daily doses of insulin—one in the morning and one in the evening.

He says he learned a lesson unrelated to diabetes. "You've got to go to the bathroom very quickly" to avoid dangerous exposure to the temperatures and wind.

On days when the journey felt impossible, Cross admits to experiencing some doubt.

"A few times, [Cross and his traveling partner] asked ourselves, 'what the hell are we doing out here?'"

He says his experience as an athlete has helped him understand that some days are harder than others.

"You build that into your training and your mental planning process," Cross explains. "You know you're going to have days like that. Then, when you have one, you just keep getting on with it. It's like having diabetes; there's no point in complaining. You've got diabetes, whether you complain about it or not. Just get on with it."

Cross says that, over the course of the trip, his heart rate adjusted to the extreme exertion and his body's energy expenditure to keep warm. Nearly 140 beats per minute at the outset, by the time they reached the South Pole his heart rate fell to 112.

Sixty-one days after they set out, on January 17, Cross and his travel partner arrived at the South Pole.

"I think these expeditions are directly applicable to many parts of my life," says Cross. "It's similar to having diabetes; you've got to plan, prepare, and execute."

— Expert Commentary —

In 1921, a surgeon at the University of Toronto named Frederick Banting and his assistant Charles Best were successfully able to extract insulin from a dog's pancreas. With this concoction they were able to keep another dog with diabetes alive for 70 days. Along with colleagues John Macleod and biochemist James B. Collip, the group was able to extract a purer form of insulin from the pancreas of cattle. This concoction was injected in January 1922 into a 14-year-old boy named Leonard Thompson, who was dying from diabetes. Thompson went on to live until 1935 because of the amazing discovery of insulin. Banting and Macleod were jointly awarded the Nobel Prize in Medicine in 1923, and they shared the prize with other members of the research team.

Fast forward over 80 years and the accomplishments of Will Cross become even more amazing. Without insulin, Cross would quickly become sick and weak. This is not a good scenario even with a local hospital nearby, much less being hundreds of miles from civilization near the North Pole in subzero temperatures. The ability to keep his insulin from freezing was im-

perative and something Cross needed to assure for his trip to be a success. He was able to push his own limits physically but also push the limits of what can be done to keep insulin potent and usable.

You may not be hiking to the North or South Pole, but planning to keep your insulin protected is important on a hot summer day or camping out in the elements. In general, freezing insulin is not recommended. Unopened and unused insulin should be stored in the refrigerator at a temperature of 36° to 46°F. Once an insulin vial or pen is opened and in use, it should be maintained at "room temperature," typically thought of as between 56° and 80°F.

UNAFRAID TO GRAPPLE for a rebound or hit the floor chasing a loose ball, Lauren Cox, who wears both a continuous glucose monitor (CGM) and an insulin pump on the court, doesn't back down from physical play.

Cox, who says she was shy about her diabetes as a child, wears her insulin pump beneath her uniform jersey—not to hide it but to protect it from bumps, falls, and the general roughness that her on-court position requires.

"It can definitely get physical under the basket," she says.

The CGM is about the size of a silver dollar and holds a sensor and a transmitter. When a person attaches a CGM, a small filament pierces the skin, allowing the sensor access to the wearer's interstitial fluid. The glucose level in the interstitial fluid is similar to glucose levels in the blood, but there may be a short time lag. Every few minutes, the real-time sensor checks interstitial fluid glucose levels and the transmitter sends that information back to a handheld device or a smartphone. The data can be useful in learning what foods or activities drive sugars too high or too low. The wearer can analyze trends and make adjustments to nutrition or routine.

Most CGMs reduce or eliminate the need for finger sticks and,

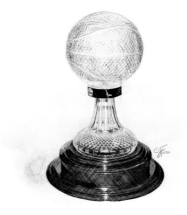

NCAA women's basketball trophy

because they test levels so frequently, can provide a full picture of the ups and downs of a wearer's blood glucose.

Cox's CGM tends to get some pretty tough wear. During her years at Baylor, Cox was a frequent target of double-teaming defenses. At 6 feet, 4 inches tall, she's a scoring and passing threat near the basket. Defenses collapse hard on her, which means a lot of swinging elbows and some rough play.

Cox affixes her CGM to the back of one of her upper arms and typically uses two kinds of tape to keep it attached and safe from flying elbows. She covers the monitor with a few wraps of athletic tape, then covers that with a flex wrap. Fans who don't know she has diabetes wouldn't notice anything out of the ordinary about a player who wears tape around one of her muscular arms.

"Sometimes my monitor gets bumped around," she says. When on-court jostling knocks the sensor out of Cox's skin, she yanks off the tape and the CGM and flings them toward her team's bench.

"I've had to rip it off and throw it to the sideline once or twice."

From time to time, Cox experiences low blood sugar during her team's practices. She takes a short break, slugs down some fruit juice, and within minutes feels well enough to return to practice.

Now and then, like nearly everyone with diabetes, Cox experiences hypoglycemia, even when she follows her regular routine. She remembers a game day during her freshman season at Baylor when her blood sugar was too high for her to play.

She sticks closely to her game-day routines, which helps keep her blood sugar in normal ranges.

"I eat the same things every game day. I do the same things an hour, two hours before every game," she says. "I find that works better for me than going back and looking at the data [from her CGM]."

Game days at Baylor involved a light practice and shoot-around early in the day, says Cox. The team ate its meals four hours before tip-off.

"Grilled chicken, some fruit, vegetables, and a roll," she says. "And water. That's my meal before every game."

When her team arrived at the arena two hours prior to game time, Cox had a granola bar and a sports drink before warmups.

"Then right before the game, I check my blood sugar to make sure it's in that 100 to 120 [mg/dl] range," she says. "Sometimes during the warmups, my sugar drops. So, I'll drink an apple juice."

— *Expert Commentary* —

Having a routine can be helpful for many people with diabetes. Eating the same meals every day is common, and often special considerations to manage blood glucose during training is needed (Box 6.2). Many people who exercise tend to do the same types of workouts routinely. These behaviors allow individuals with diabetes to better anticipate how their blood sugars will respond to certain scenarios from prior experience. Lauren Cox's pregame meal and regimen is a good example of this. She had honed her "diabetes skills," similar to her basketball skills, to know how she would respond to her pregame meal done at a similar time before her game coupled with her snacks and warmups. This type of routine typically helps.

BOX 6.2
Blood Glucose Management during and after Exercise

Planning meals and insulin dosing around exercise can be a challenge. Some basic guiding principles can be helpful.

1. Exercised muscles are more sensitive to insulin. This leads to greater glucose lowering for a given amount of insulin *after* exercise compared to when someone has not exercised. For example, consider two consecutive Sunday afternoons. On the first Sunday you lounge on the couch all day watching football. The most activity you do is to hop up and cheer your team scoring a touchdown. The following Sunday afternoon you head to the golf course and walk 18 holes. Both Sunday nights you sit down for the same meal with a starting glucose of 150 md/dl. You dose 5 units of insulin and eat the meal each time, but your glucose values are vastly different at bedtime on these consecutive Sundays. Your glucose is 215 md/dl at bedtime following your day of watching football compared to 78 md/dl at bedtime following your round of golf. This example shows how exercise can markedly affect your response to insulin.

2. Reduced insulin doses may be needed following exercise, such as bolusing less aggressively for meals or snacks after exercise. Basal insulin injection reductions after exercise or a temporary reduced basal rate on an insulin pump may be needed for a few hours after exercise.

3. After intense exercise, a small snack may be necessary at bedtime with no insulin to help prevent overnight hypoglycemia.

4. Hybrid closed loop insulin pumps and sensors offer the option to inform the algorithm that you are exercising. This allows the system to target a higher glucose while in the "exercise mode" and help prevent post-exercise hypoglycemia.

As reflected in the stories of these athletes on training and competition days, sometimes things don't go as planned and understanding this can sometimes happen will help prevent frustration. There are many factors that play a role in blood glucose that we can't always account for, such as stress, fatigue, and acute illness to name a few. It is important to be prepared and have a routine to minimize unpredictable fluctuations in blood glucose.

Chapter 7

Building a Community
How can I give back?

BY THE TIME ADAM DRISCOLL and his friends decided to ride fixed-gear bicycles across the United States, Driscoll was something of an old hand at the feat. He'd ridden in eight-, four-, and two-man teams in the Race Across America, an annual competition where cycling teams pedal from Pacific to Atlantic.

But the Adventures For the Cure ride wasn't a race. And while it did begin on one side of the United States and end on the other, it was more than a cross-country ride.

A year or so before their cross-country odyssey, Driscoll and his roommate Pat Blair started a nonprofit organization to bring attention to type 1 diabetes and to raise money for research into curing the disease. College pals Driscoll, who was diagnosed with type 1 at age 12, and Blair had post-college jobs that paid the bills. But both felt compelled to do a little more with their lives.

Started in 2006, Adventures For the Cure (AFC) has previously raised hundreds of thousands of dollars for a camp in Cecil County, Maryland, dedicated to providing children who have type 1 diabetes a supportive and fun camp experience and raises awareness for diabetes.

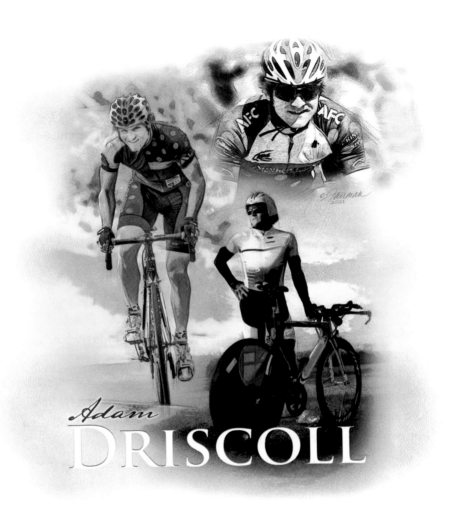

Adam

DRISCOLL

Adam Driscoll, American cyclist and former member of a four-man relay team that rode in the world's longest bicycle race, the Race Across America: *"For them to see that here I am, riding across the country with diabetes and it's not stopping me. That's the impression I was trying to make."*

A few years prior to their 2012 journey—which began in Washington state, meandered around the country, and ended in Ocean City, Maryland—Driscoll had raced across the United States with Team Type 1. The racers rarely stopped, slept in vans, and generally pushed as hard as they could toward the finish line.

As the AFC riders crossed America, they stopped and connected with people. Driscoll, Blair, two other riders, and their van crew made friends wherever they went. They paid particular attention to making friends with kids who have diabetes.

Driscoll says his own childhood diagnosis went about as smoothly as it could go. But even an outgoing kid like him felt the need to hide the fact that he had diabetes from his friends. He took pains to test his blood sugar in private, afraid other kids would think he was weird.

"I think a lot of kids are like I was," he says. "They struggle to hide that they have diabetes. I want them to know that it's not anything to feel ashamed of."

On the AFC ride, Driscoll connected with two kids with whom he's still in touch.

Tess, a 12-year-old from Iowa who had been diagnosed recently with type 1 diabetes, had a little adventure of her own with Driscoll. As the AFC guys rolled through her state, Tess joined Driscoll on a tandem bike for a 30-mile stretch.

With Driscoll, decked out in his full AFC cycling kit, up front, Tess pedaled the bike's rear wheel with her pink bicycle helmet strapped tightly on her head. Before the ride, Driscoll and Tess discussed diabetes and some of the challenges it can present for a kid. He says he saw in Tess some of the same fears and insecurities he had after his diagnosis.

"Tess was easy to talk to," says Driscoll. "She'd only just been diagnosed. I tried to somehow get across that it's OK that she has [diabetes]. I have it too."

During their tandem ride, they continued their discussion.

"That was really cool," Driscoll recalls. "It was just me and her for, like, 30 miles. I think she enjoyed it."

During their time together, including while on the tandem bike, Driscoll made a point of checking his blood sugar a few times.

"I think it was good for Tess to see me check my sugar out in public," he says. "I wanted her to know that there's nothing weird or different about her. It's normal. It's just one more thing we have to do. It's a regular routine, like brushing your teeth."

When the AFC got to Kansas City, Driscoll also connected with a newly diagnosed 5-year-old boy and his parents. Because Max was so young, Driscoll spent more time talking with the boy's parents.

"I think Max got it," says Driscoll. "But really, the focus was more on his mom and dad. At first, it can be a struggle when a kid gets diagnosed. They're the ones who have to learn it. And there's a lot to learn."

Driscoll wanted Max's parents to see that their child's diabetes doesn't have to limit him as he grows up.

"For them to see that here I am, riding across the country with diabetes and it's not stopping me. That's the impression I was trying to make."

He says he and Tess have stayed in touch, encouraging each other about their common disease and about staying active. He also still communicates with Max's parents.

"We met a lot of great people on that ride," he says. "I made some friends that I'm still friends with."

— *Expert Commentary* —

Being self-conscious about a diagnosis of diabetes is common and understandable. People worry how they will be received at school, socially, or in the workplace. Each situation is unique and individual, but in general people with diabetes find their concerns of how they will be viewed regarding their diag-

nosis to be unwarranted. Talking to classmates, teachers, friends, coworkers, or teammates about what diabetes is, how it is treated, and separating fact from fiction can make transparency with diabetes much easier. If peers are educated about the disease, they are more willing to help, understand, and support. In general, lack of knowledge about diabetes and a misunderstanding of the disease by peers is what leads to problems. Again, every situation is different and unique. Being up front and open about a diagnosis may not be something people are comfortable with from the start. But using education for peers and sharing what living with diabetes is like typically leads to comfort and ease with being open about the disease.

"SOMETHING I REALLY LOVE to do is to talk to kids who are struggling with their diabetes," says Mark Andrews of the NFL's Baltimore Ravens. "The kids and their families both need to be involved. It's going to be part of life."

The Pro Bowl tight end has an important message for people with diabetes.

"Don't let diabetes define you," he urges. "Understand your disease and understand your body. Diabetes is a part of you. But it's not who you are."

As Andrews developed into an elite professional athlete, he paid close attention to the effects the disease had on his body: what and when to eat, how much insulin he needs, when to push hard, and when to rest.

"I saw my endocrinologist every three months since I was a kid," Andrews says. "It helped that my dad is a doctor. But even kids whose parents aren't medical professionals can do what I did. I just got into healthy habits when I was young and I've stuck with them."

Andrews knows that diabetes can be an isolating disease. It can sometimes feel like you're the only person in the world who has to pay attention to managing glucose. He urges kids who have diabetes to rely on their family and friends for help.

"Surround yourself with people who care about you and who have your best interests at heart," he advises. "There will always be challenges and complications that come along with diabetes. But as long as you have those people to look after you, everything's going to be OK."

Major league pitcher Jason Johnson has a message similar to Andrews's.

When Johnson played for the Baltimore Orioles, he was a frequent visitor to the city's two major children's hospitals. Over his five seasons in the city, Johnson established himself as a big-league starting pitcher and as a person devoted to helping others.

But when he signed with the Detroit Tigers for the 2004 season, Johnson began wearing an insulin pump on the field. Clipped to the back of his belt, the device was small but easy for fans to spot.

"That's when the letters started to pour in," he says. "They said things like, 'my son has type 1 diabetes and he noticed that you have an insulin pump.' I ended up inviting a lot of different kids down to the field at Comerica Park. During batting practice, we'd talk about dealing with diabetes and stuff like that."

As the first player to wear an insulin pump on the field during a major league game, Johnson wants kids with diabetes to know that they're not alone.

"I think it helped kids to see a baseball player with the same disease they have," he says. "I just wanted them to know that, 'hey, you're OK. It doesn't have to limit you. You're just as good as everybody else.'"

Johnson remembers what his parents told him when he was 11, after his doctor told him there would be things that diabetes would prevent him from doing.

"My dad and mom sat me down," he recalls. "And my dad said, 'Look, Jason. Don't take this to mean you're done. Don't listen to what the doctors are telling you. You can do anything you want in life. You want to be a baseball player? Then go be a baseball player. Stick with it.' That's still the best advice anyone's ever given me."

He says his parents' advice is the reason he's still encouraging children with diabetes to pursue their dreams.

"There might be some kids whose parents aren't as supportive as mine were," says Johnson. "So, baseball has allowed me to kind of help and maybe teach them the same thing I was taught."

— Expert Commentary —

Mark Andrews's comments about surrounding yourself with people who care about you and have your best interest at heart rings so true in people who thrive with their diabetes. Friends and family who believe in you and your dreams are vitally important. Diabetes provides challenges at each phase of life. Having friends and family there to help you through the hard times and support you with successes and failures is crucial. It can take a team of people to succeed with diabetes; you don't have to do it all by yourself. Finding a health care provider who you trust and who is supportive is important as well, as illustrated by Jason Johnson's experiences in his early years. Explain your goals to that provider and hopefully you can form a winning team that helps you achieve your dreams in school, work, athletics, and life. If the team is not working, don't be afraid to seek out another provider who may be better able to advise you.

"NO ONE HAD EVER competed in the Olympics with diabetes before" his medal-earning performance in the 2000 Sydney

BOX 7.1
Nonprofit Organizations for Diabetes

If you have diabetes, making use of all available resources to support your disease can be extremely helpful. Local and national organizations offer guidance and support to newly diagnosed patients and those with long-standing disease. Below are a few of these organizations; there are also many others. Talk with your health care provider about available options where you live.

- *AACE Prescription Affordability Resource Center* (**prescription help.aace.com**): This site is run by the American Association of Clinical Endocrinologists. It aggregates available information and resources on patient assistance programs to help make diabetes medicines affordable to those with financial limitations.

- *American Diabetes Association* (**diabetes.org**): This national organization with local chapters supports all types of patients with diabetes. It educates patients and providers about diabetes. It funds research to manage, prevent, and cure diabetes. The ADA website is an excellent resource for dietary advice and basic diabetes education.

- *Beyond Type 1 and Beyond Type 2* (**beyondtype1.org and beyondtype2.org**): Beyond Type 1 focuses on education, advocacy, and a pathway to cures for Type 1 diabetes. Beyond Type 2 is focused on helping those with type 2 diabetes to find a community of support with education resources.

- *DiabetesSisters* (**diabetessisters.org**): This organization offers education and support for women with diabetes to help them

Games, Gary Hall Jr. says. His primary care physician and other doctors to whom he spoke were convinced that diabetes and Olympic-level swimming were not a good match.

But finding a diabetes specialist who understood his drive to compete helped to lessen his burden. Hall says his endocrinologist didn't give him a pep talk or an inspirational speech when she agreed to take him on as a patient.

live healthier and fuller lives. It offers peer support groups for women, as well as many other resources and webinars online, and advocates on their behalf.

- *The diaTribe Foundation* (**diatribe.org/foundation**): This organization was founded to improve the lives of people with diabetes and to advocate for action. It has resources to help patients make sense of their diabetes through its patient-focused online publication.

- *Endocrine Society* (**endocrine.org/patient-engagement**): The Endocrine Society is the largest organization of endocrinologists in the world and provides endocrine-related patient guides, Q&A fact sheets, and tracking logs. Patient outreach initiatives bring medical experts to diverse communities. The physician referral directory helps patients to find an endocrinologist.

- **JDRF (JDRF.org):** This national organization with local chapters focuses on patients with type 1 diabetes. It offers support such as on-call volunteers to contact with questions, one-on-one mentoring for newly diagnosed patients, and community forums. Care kits are provided for newly diagnosed patients—tailored to children, teens, or adults. In addition, JDRF raises money to support research focused on type 1 diabetes.

- *Take Control of Your Diabetes* (**TCOYD.org**): This organization offers education in the form of conferences, videos, newsletters, and more to patients with diabetes and their family members. It also works to educate health care providers who care for patients with diabetes.

"She just said, 'Well, it hasn't been done before. But let's give it a try.' And a year and a half later, after making the right changes to my training, I was back in the pool at the Olympics."

He brought home four medals from Sydney: a bronze, a silver, and two golds.

For several years after his swimming career ended, Hall maintained a nonprofit organization he started. The organization raised

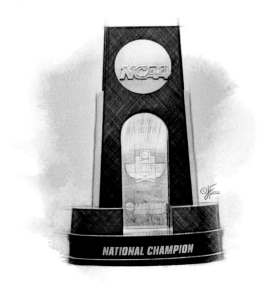

NCAA women's lacrosse national champion trophy

money to support research of type 1 diabetes. But it also paid for supplies for underserved kids with the disease. He continues to serve as an advocate for people with type 1 diabetes.

Raising money to fund diabetes research can be a great way to support people with the disease. Since 2015, the University of Maryland women's lacrosse team has hosted an annual type 1 diabetes awareness game, in honor of Riley Reese, son of Terps head coach Cathy Reese. The games have raised over $50,000 for type 1 diabetes research. The team wears special jerseys for the game and sells replicas online and at the stadium.

"It's pretty cool that we're able to raise money" for research, Reese says. "I remember one year, I connected with a mom on the sidelines whose really young son was just diagnosed. It's been good."

Reese says, since Riley's diagnosis, she has talked to many parents whose kids have diabetes.

"After we learned that Riley has it, we just had to read about and learn about a lot of stuff ourselves," she says. If she can pass along some of the knowledge she's gained as a mom, Reese says she's glad to do it.

"A lot of it was figuring out how we were going to manage and make Riley's life as normal as possible," Reese recalls. "So, I like being able to share what we've learned."

— Expert Commentary —

The affordability of medications and supplies for diabetes remains a concern in many parts of the world, including the United States, where the price of newer insulins has skyrocketed over recent decades and the cost of glucose strips, in particular, has led many patients to ration insulin or re-use test strips. Organizations that support patients with diabetes, such as the one founded by Hall, are important to ensure that they are able to access the health care they need. There are many large nonprofit organizations for diabetes in the United States (Box 7.1) and around the world. These organizations depend on individuals such as Reese to fundraise, volunteer, or contribute in other ways to achieve their mission and can be an impactful way to be involved in the larger diabetes community. Though said often, it cannot be said enough: one person can make a difference. Sharing personal stories with those who are navigating a similar experience can be invaluable, especially with a new diagnosis of diabetes.

CYCLIST MONIQUE HANLEY started an organization in her native Australia dedicated to encouraging people with diabetes to get active. Part of her focus these days is a campaign aimed at modernizing the exercise guidelines for people who have the disease.

Too often, Hanley says, exercise guidelines for both children and

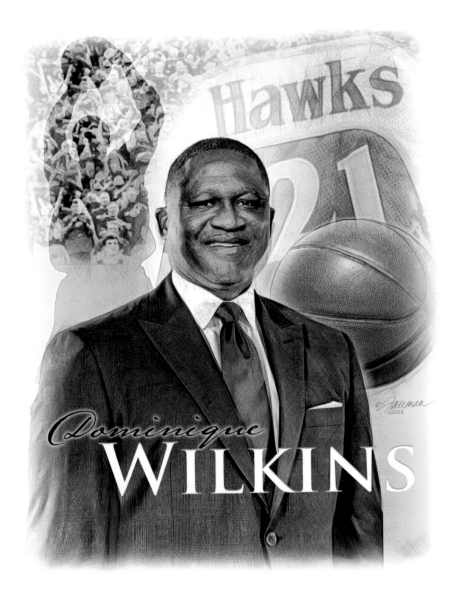

Dominique Wilkins, American basketball Hall of Famer and president of basketball for the National Basketball Association's Atlanta Hawks: *"I just think of [diabetes] as another opponent I compete with."*

adults fail to account for the disease's complexities. As an example, Hanley asserts that one glucose reading, with no context, is a poor way to dictate whether or not a kid can handle physical exertion.

"One test is arbitrary," she says. "To know what's really going on, you need two tests, at least 10 minutes apart. We need two data points to see a trend. If you say a student can't exercise with a glucose level of, say, 270, you don't know whether that number is going up or down. You're not considering whether there's insulin on board. It's a completely uninformed guideline, and it really doesn't help anyone."

Hanley is working to get state and national health officials in Australia to adopt more comprehensive, better-informed guidelines for exercising with diabetes.

"It's really just about smarter risk management," says Hanley, who in addition to working to bring attention to diabetes and physical activity, also serves as an outspoken activist in the area of women's athletics in Australia.

Like Hanley, basketball Hall of Famer Dominique Wilkins uses his notoriety to encourage people to get active and to get screened.

Wilkins was diagnosed with type 2 diabetes at age 40. His outreach is typically aimed more in the direction of adults with type 2 or with prediabetes, particularly African Americans, who are disproportionately diagnosed with type 2 diabetes.

"I told myself that I have to find ways to not just help myself," he says, "but to help educate other people about healthier options."

Wilkins is a spokesperson for a large pharmaceutical company that makes and sells diabetes-related products, from insulin to medicines that stimulate the body to produce its own insulin. He regularly speaks to people about the importance of getting tested for diabetes.

"Screenings tell you whether something's wrong," he says. "If you don't know what's wrong, you can't do much about it. And believe me—if you ignore diabetes, it'll bite you.

"I tell people, just get up and get moving."

— Expert Commentary —

The exercise guidelines for individuals with type 1 or type 2 diabetes from the American Diabetes Association include a minimum of 150 minutes of moderate to vigorous aerobic exercise per week, spread over at least three days during the week, with no more than two days in a row without activity. According to the American Heart Association, this includes activities such as brisk walking (at least 2.5 miles per hour), dancing, gardening, heavy yardwork, swimming, tennis, hiking, running, bicycling, or jumping rope. A few bouts of muscle-strengthening activity (such as resistance or weights) during the week and decreased sedentary time is also recommended. However, these guidelines can be challenging to integrate into a busy daily schedule. Starting with small changes, such as walking instead of driving or taking the stairs instead of the elevator, may be easier to implement. Healthier neighborhoods that promote walkability can provide opportunities for people to be physically active. The Centers for Disease Control and Prevention (CDC) has initiatives to help neighborhoods promote walkability; examples include adding safer sidewalks, pedestrian crossings, and protected bike lanes.

WHEN STAR SOFTBALL PLAYER Kylee Perez graduated from UCLA, she knew just what her next step would be. She applied to graduate schools in southern California and is on her way to becoming a nurse.

"When I was first diagnosed, I had the most amazing nurses," she says. "That's why I want to be a nurse—so I can do for other people what they did for me."

Perez says her nurses helped her keep a positive outlook on life with diabetes.

"I cannot thank them enough."

BOX 7.2
Depression and Diabetes

Depression is a common disorder causing a persistent feeling of sadness or loss of interest in your usual activities. People with depression often have difficulty with normal day-to-day activities like sleeping, eating, or working. Unfortunately, people with diabetes are twice as likely to be afflicted with depression as those without diabetes. If you are struggling with depression, diabetes becomes much more difficult to control. Often, you need to get control your depression before you can take control of your diabetes. Here are some helpful tips to keep in mind:

- Feeling sad or blue every now and then can be very normal. Depression goes beyond this.

- People who are depressed have some of the following symptoms nearly every day for two weeks or more: fatigue, concentration problems, irritability, feelings of hopelessness, weight loss, loss of appetite, sleep problems, and loss of interest in usual activities.

- If you think you are suffering from depression, talk to your diabetes provider about it. This may not otherwise come up during a short office visit. But by bringing it up and taking steps to address it, this can make you feel better and improve your diabetes!

- There are many treatment options available for depression. The most common are cognitive behavioral therapy and drug therapy.

- Cognitive behavioral therapy is sometimes called "talk therapy." You work with a therapist or psychologist who is trained to help you better deal with depression by approaching challenges in your life differently.

- Drug therapy includes a wide array of available medications that can treat depression.

- If you end up taking antidepressant medications, it is important to recognize that many don't work overnight. Talk to your health care provider about the specifics of your medication but know that many of these medicines take a few weeks to start fully working.

- If you are on antidepressant medications and experience side effects (like fatigue, dry mouth, or an upset stomach), don't just stop the medicine on your own. Let your health care provider know so they can work with you to find other treatment options.

During her years at UCLA, Perez talked with many newly diagnosed kids. It was common for parents to email Perez, explaining that a young son or daughter had type 1 diabetes. Despite her busy athletic and academic schedules, Perez always made time to talk to kids and parents, encouraging them to stay positive and avoid feelings that diabetes should place any limits on them.

Some of the best, most important encouragement a newly diagnosed person can get is from other people with diabetes.

Long-jump athlete Kate Hall-Harnden has a message similar to Perez's for the kids she meets. But since track and field meets don't typically draw large crowds in the United States, she has spoken mostly with people in Europe.

"Track is huge there," she says. "At meets in Europe, there's all kinds of people waiting for an autograph or a picture. It's great, because I'm really passionate about telling my story and letting people know that diabetes doesn't have to stop anyone from doing anything."

Being a track athlete can be an expensive proposition, especially when you're not part of a team, like Hall-Harnden. Sponsorships offset the costs of travel and training. One of Hall-Harnden's sponsors is a company that makes and sells the insulin pump she prefers.

"That's a good opportunity to talk to people," she says. "Sometimes I'll speak for Omnipod and share my story that way."

— *Expert Commentary* —

Maintaining a positive outlook is vital when dealing with the challenges that may arise from having a chronic disease such as diabetes. It is not uncommon to feel overwhelmed or be discouraged, worried, frustrated, or tired of dealing with daily diabetes care—this is often referred to as diabetes distress. However, it is important to not let unpredictable trials and tribulations get you down; talking to your health care provider or seeing a mental health counselor, if needed, can be helpful. In some individuals, a persistently low mood, withdrawal, apathy, or irritability may indicate signs of depression

(Box 7.2). Clinical depression may result in difficulties sleeping, eating more or less than usual, sedentary behavior, and an overall decreased motivation to self-manage diabetes at home. People with diabetes are much more likely than others to have depression. Seeking medical advice for diagnosis and treatment of depression when present is important not only for personal well-being but also to ensure that diabetes is optimally managed.

BODYBUILDING CHAMPION DOUG BURNS has been a regular speaker at type 1 diabetes conferences like the annual Friends for Life meeting held every summer in Orlando, Florida. Kids and their families travel to the conference from around the country to connect with each other, share diabetes management tips, listen to diabetes doctors, and hear encouraging words from speakers like Burns.

The former Natural Mr. Universe recalls a Friends for Life conference he attended with Chris Dudley, who played 16 seasons in the NBA and also has type 1 diabetes. Waiting for the beginning of a session where Burns and Dudley were to speak to a group of 40 or so kids with diabetes, the two athletes made some small talk about their struggles with hypoglycemia.

"I was surprised that Chris had some of the same troubles I'd had with low blood sugar," Burns says.

They compared some experiences, shared a few tips and, before long, it was time for the session to begin. Burns kicked off the session by asking for a show of hands:

"How many of you here today sometimes have trouble with low blood sugar?"

No hands went up. Burns figured it must be a group of children with extraordinarily well-managed diabetes. Impressive, he thought.

As the session went on, Burns and Dudley shared their stories of training, competing, and winning, despite living with diabetes. As they spoke, a few stragglers joined the session 5 or 10 minutes late.

At the end, when the speakers opened the floor for questions, one of the late-arriving kids raised his hand. Burns guesses the boy was about 12.

"He asked the first question," Burns remembered. "He said, 'Do either of you ever have problems with hypoglycemia?'"

Because the boy had arrived a few minutes late, he hadn't heard Burns ask the group the same question.

"I looked over at Chris Dudley and he was smiling," says Burns. "I told the boy that Chris and I had just been talking about that before the session started. And yes, we both fight low blood sugar, the same as you."

After Burns and Dudley finished addressing the boy's question, Burns again asked for a show of hands.

"OK, let's try this again," he said to the group. "*Now* how many of you have had trouble with hypoglycemia?"

Burns says every hand in the room went up.

"Every single kid in that room had experience with low blood sugar," he says. "But they didn't raise their hands the first time I asked. It was a reminder of how self-conscious and tentative kids can be about sharing their experiences with diabetes, even in a roomful of other kids who have it. It took one brave kid to break the ice for everybody."

— *Expert Commentary* —

Bravery can come in many forms, such as the courage of a young child who speaks up to share his challenges with others. Reaching out to others and learning from those who have navigated the same disease are often important first steps in building a community. By offering their personal stories of how they have thrived while living with diabetes, and the worthy initiatives they have undertaken to give back to the community, the professional athletes and their families featured in this book offer an unprecedented window into the common experiences that all individuals living with diabetes may encounter in their day-to-day lives. Thank you to the athletes for taking these bold steps in shaping the diabetes community.

If readers take away one thing from this book, the authors would like it to be this: you're never alone. There are communities of people who are living and thriving with diabetes, and they're a great resource for information, for ideas, and for friendship. And there are people in every field who are examples of how to live well, while also managing a chronic disease such as diabetes.

Index

Page numbers in *italics* refer to images.

tubed, 50, 51; tubeless, 50, 51; using, 51; wearing during exercise, 83, 130, 146–47, 156
insulin resistance: after exercise, 128; and body fat, 77; described, 27; and dietary fat, 47; and losing weight, 44; and prediabetes, 4, 10–11; and Type 2 diabetes, 4, 10–11, 33, 114
insulin sensitivity: and exertion, 101, 108, 149; and insulin pumps, 51
insulin therapy: basal insulin, 28–29, 51, 122, 149; bolus insulin, 51, 122, 149; carbohydrates ratio, 43–44, 51; cost of, 161; development of, 64, 145; effect of fat on, 47–48; and initial treatment after diagnosis, 13, 14; mechanisms of, 10; rationing of, 161; storage during activities, 94, 140; storage temperatures, 54, 90, 140, 143, 145–46; and Type 2 diabetes, 11, 28, 44, 114; types of, 121, 122. *See also* glucose monitoring; insulin, injectable; insulin pens; insulin pumps
interval training, 128
intestinal motility, 47
Ironman Triathlons, 59–60
islets, 27

JDRF organization, 159
Johnson, Jason, xii, 45–47, 101–4, *102*, 131–32, 156–57
Jones, Coburn, 101
juice, 22, 54, 75, 97
juvenile diabetes. *See* diabetes, Type 1

kidney complications, 38, 39, 78
Kimball, Charlie, xii, 7–10, *8*, 21–24

lacrosse: NCAA Women's Lacrosse trophy, *160. See also* Reese, Riley

learning: in athletes' stories, 21–22, 28–31, 34–39, 40–42, 55, 61, 68–69; by coaches and teammates, 29–30, 34, 99–104, 129–30; and DSMES training, 71; and initial diagnosis, 13; and monitors, 68, 71, 146; by parents, 12–14, 95, 154; resources on, 71; and self-management, 34, 61, 65, 66, 68–69, 71, 72, 92, 101
Libre sensor, 52
lightheadedness, 23
linagliptin, 112
lipohypertrophy, 134
liraglutide, 112
liver, 78
lixisenatide, 112

Macleod, John, 145
management. *See* glucose monitoring; self-management
medications: contraindications for, 112; costs of, 161; for depression, 165; and DSMES training, 71; non-insulin medications, 23, 28, 112, 114; resources on, 158; and routine preventive care, 78; side effects, 112, 122; sulfonylureas, 23, 28, 112
Medtronic, 52
meglitinides, 112
metformin, 112
miglitol, 112
MLB World Series Championship Trophy, 46
monitoring. *See* glucose monitoring
monosaccharides, 10. *See also* glucose
mountaineering. *See* Cross, Will; Sasseville, Sébastien
Mr. Olympia bodybuilding trophy, *37*
Mulkey, Kim, 30
muscle growth and insulin, 92
muscle-strengthening exercise, 79, 128

About the Authors

Mark D. Corriere, MD. Dr. Corriere worked as a general internist in the United States Navy for over a decade, where he proudly treated active-duty service members, retirees, and their family members. Following his navy career, he completed fellowship training in Endocrinology, Diabetes, and Metabolism at Johns Hopkins University School of Medicine. He is currently a clinical endocrinologist at Maryland Endocrine in Columbia, Maryland, where he treats adults with all types of diabetes. He also is a coauthor of the award-winning book *Diabetes Head to Toe: Everything You Need to Know about Diagnosis, Treatment, and Living with Diabetes*. Dr. Corriere is a past president of the Maryland Endocrine and Metabolism Society. An avid endurance runner and youth sports coach, he has also completed several marathons and ultramarathons. In addition to his family and diabetes, he is passionate about Notre Dame football and Baltimore Orioles baseball.

Rita R. Kalyani, MD, MHS. Dr. Kalyani is an associate professor of Medicine at Johns Hopkins University School of Medicine in the Division of Endocrinology, Diabetes, and Metabolism and a nationally recognized thought leader, researcher, and clinician in diabetes who is actively involved in diabetes education and public awareness initiatives. She holds an undergraduate degree from Harvard College and completed her medical degree, residency, and fellowship at Johns Hopkins. Dr. Kalyani's clinical practice is based in the Johns Hopkins Comprehensive Diabetes Center. She is the editor in chief of the Johns Hopkins Patient Guide to Diabetes website. An author of more than 125 peer-reviewed research publications, Dr. Kalyani's research has been funded by the National Institutes of Health and focuses on diabetes and its complications in high-risk populations. She is a past chair of the American Diabetes Association's Professional Practice Committee, which oversees all of the organization's clinical practice guidelines. Dr. Kalyani is also a coauthor of the award-winning book, *Diabetes Head to Toe: Everything You Need to Know about Diagnosis, Treatment, and Living with Diabetes*, published by Johns Hopkins University Press.

Patrick J. Smith. Mr. Smith is a biomedical science writer at Johns Hopkins University School of Medicine, where he covers clinical and research breakthroughs for the Division of Endocrinology, Diabetes, and Metabolism, as well as the Division of Gastroenterology and Hepatology. A former newspaper reporter and speechwriter for various elected officials, Mr. Smith is the author of *Extra Innings: The Joy and the Pains of Over-30 Baseball*, published by McFarland in 2007. From 2007 through 2018, he served as a writer, then managing editor of the baseball-writing websites BugsAndCranks.com and TheSpitter.com. He lives in Baltimore, Maryland.